Yoga

Recent Titles in
Q&A Health Guides

Substance Abuse: Your Questions Answered
Romeo Vitelli

Eating Disorders: Your Questions Answered
Justine J. Reel

Food Allergies and Sensitivities: Your Questions Answered
Alice C. Richer

Obesity: Your Questions Answered
Christine L. B. Selby

Birth Control: Your Questions Answered
Paul Quinn

Therapy and Counseling: Your Questions Answered
Christine L. B. Selby

Depression: Your Questions Answered
Romeo Vitelli

Food Labels: Your Questions Answered
Barbara A. Brehm

Smoking: Your Questions Answered
Stacy Mintzer Herlihy

Grief and Loss: Your Questions Answered
Louis Kuykendall Jr.

Teen Stress: Your Questions Answered
Nicole Neda Zamanzadeh and Tamara D. Afifi

Healthy Friendships: Your Questions Answered
Lauren Holleb

Trauma and Resilience: Your Questions Answered
Keith A. Young

Vegetarian and Vegan Diets: Your Questions Answered
Alice C. Richer

YOGA

Your Questions Answered

Anjali A. Sarkar

Q&A Health Guides

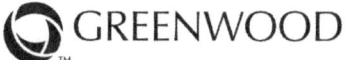

An Imprint of ABC-CLIO, LLC
Santa Barbara. California • Denver. Colorado

Library of Congress Cataloging-in-Publication Data

Names: Sarkar, Anjali A., author.
Title: Yoga : your questions answered / Anjali A. Sarkar.
Description: First Edition. | Santa Barbara : ABC-CLIO, 2021. | Series: Q&a
  health guides | Includes bibliographical references and index.
Identifiers: LCCN 2020035101 (print) | LCCN 2020035102 (ebook) | ISBN
  9781440871726 (hardcover) | ISBN 9781440871733 (ebook)
Subjects: LCSH: Hatha yoga for teenagers. | Hatha yoga—Miscellanea. |
  Self-care, Health.
Classification: LCC RA781.7 .S263 2021 (print) | LCC RA781.7 (ebook) |
  DDC 613.7/046—dc23
LC record available at https://lccn.loc.gov/2020035101
LC ebook record available at https://lccn.loc.gov/2020035102

ISBN: 978-1-4408-7172-6 (print)
        978-1-4408-7173-3 (ebook)

25 24 23 22 21   1 2 3 4 5

This book is also available as an eBook.

Greenwood
An Imprint of ABC-CLIO, LLC

ABC-CLIO, LLC
147 Castilian Drive
Santa Barbara, California 93117
www.abc-clio.com

This book is printed on acid-free paper ∞

Manufactured in the United States of America

For my mother and first yoga teacher, Bharati Roy-Sarkar

Contents

Series Foreword   xi

Acknowledgments   xiii

Introduction   xv

Guide to Health Literacy   xvii

Common Misconceptions about Yoga   xxv

Questions and Answers   1

General Information   3

  1. What is yoga?   3
  2. Is yoga a religion? Do I have to follow a certain
     religion to do yoga?   4
  3. What do some of the Sanskrit words used in yoga class
     mean, like "Namaste" and "Om/Aum"? Is it necessary
     for me to remember the names of poses?   6
  4. What is pranayama?   9
  5. When and where did people first begin practicing yoga,
     and when did it come to the United States?   11
  6. What are the different types of yoga?   13
  7. Are there scientific or medical studies that show the
     efficacy of yoga?   18

Benefits 21

8. Why should I practice yoga? 21
9. How can yoga help me find balance in life? 23
10. I'm an insomniac. Can yoga help me sleep better? 27
11. I have ADHD. Can yoga help me cope better? 29
12. How can yoga help me get better grades? 31
13. Which yoga poses treat adrenal fatigue and chronic stress? 32
14. Which poses prevent lower back pain? 33
15. Why do I feel a "yoga high" after class? 35
16. Is practicing yoga during pregnancy beneficial for delivery? 37
17. Will yoga help me get better at sports? 39
18. What impact does yoga have on flexibility? Do I need to be flexible to do yoga? 41
19. Is yoga a good way to improve muscle strength? 42
20. Is yoga beneficial for losing weight? 44

Risks and Concerns 47

21. What should I do if I feel physical discomfort or pain in a yoga pose? 47
22. Why do my joints pop during practice? 49
23. Why do I get dizzy during yoga? 50
24. Why do my muscles shake or tremble during yoga? 52
25. Why am I not supposed to eat two to three hours before yoga practice? How do I manage my diet to get maximum benefit from my yoga practice? 53
26. Is it safe to practice inversions? 54
27. Should I practice yoga if I'm on my period? 56
28. Is it safe to practice yoga after an injury? 58
29. What injuries are most likely to occur if yoga is done incorrectly? 60
30. Does greater flexibility lead to greater risk of injury? 62
31. How do I know if I'm pushing myself too hard? 63

How to Practice Yoga 67

32. How do I know what type of yoga is best for me? 67
33. How do I know I'm ready for pranayama practice? 69
34. Should I learn yoga from a book, an online course, a group class, or a private class? 71
35. What should I look for in a yoga teacher? 73
36. How do I begin, maintain, and grow my yoga practice? 74

37. How frequently should I practice yoga or take classes? 75
38. What should I wear to yoga class? 77
39. What should I eat to aid my yoga practice? 78
40. How should I sequence yoga poses in my practice? 79
41. What types of hands-on assists should I expect from
    my teacher in yoga class? 81
42. How do I respond to hands-on adjustments in a yoga class? 83
43. How can I get more comfortable sitting cross-legged?
    Can I still do yoga if I cannot sit cross-legged? 84
44. What is the best time and place to practice yoga?
    Should I practice yoga in front of a mirror? 87
45. What equipment do I need at home for my yoga practice
    and why? 89
46. Do I need to lose weight or be more flexible before
    I can start practicing yoga? 91
47. How can I get started if I'm too shy or nervous or
    physically unable to attend a group class? 93
48. How do I improve my posture using yoga? 94
49. How can I incorporate mudras into my yoga practice? 98

Case Studies 101

Glossary 117

Directory of Resources 127

Index 131

Series Foreword

All of us have questions about our health. Is this normal? Should I be doing something differently? Whom should I talk to about my concerns? And our modern world is full of answers. Thanks to the Internet, there's a wealth of information at our fingertips, from forums where people can share their personal experiences to Wikipedia articles to the full text of medical studies. But finding the right information can be an intimidating and difficult task—some sources are written at too high a level, others have been oversimplified, while still others are heavily biased or simply inaccurate.

Q&A Health Guides address the needs of readers who want accurate, concise answers to their health questions, authored by reputable and objective experts, and written in clear and easy-to-understand language. This series focuses on the topics that matter most to young adult readers, including various aspects of physical and emotional well-being as well as other components of a healthy lifestyle. These guides will also serve as a valuable tool for parents, school counselors, and others who may need to answer teens' health questions.

All books in the series follow the same format to make finding information quick and easy. Each volume begins with an essay on health literacy and why it is so important when it comes to gathering and evaluating health information. Next, the top five myths and misconceptions that surround the topic are dispelled. The heart of each guide is a collection of questions and answers, organized thematically. A selection of five case studies provides real-world examples to illuminate key concepts. Rounding out each volume are a directory of resources, glossary, and index.

It is our hope that the books in this series will not only provide valuable information but will also help guide readers toward a lifetime of healthy decision making.

Acknowledgments

I write this compilation of basic questions and answers on yoga with the sincerest gratitude to all my yoga teachers and the lineage of teachers who have gone before them. I thank my mother, Bharati Roy-Sarkar, for introducing me to yoga and motivating me to practice daily from early childhood. I thank my uncle Dayal Roy for introducing me to the therapeutic aspects of yoga. I thank John Schumacher, Doerthe Braun, and all the yoga teachers at Unity Woods, Bethesda, Maryland, for helping me refine my practice over the years. Devoting time to this project would not have been possible without the support of my wife, Carretha D. Jackson.

Introduction

The purpose of this book is to address some basic queries on yoga that might arise in the mind of a beginner student seeking to adopt the practice. In today's world of extreme stress and constant competitiveness, the practice of yoga is becoming popular across the United States as an accessible antidote. Health benefits of yoga are widely reported in medical journals and the mainstream media. According to a recent National Health Interview Survey (NHIS) reported by the National Center for Complementary and Integrative Health (NCCIH), 21 million adults and 1.7 million children practice yoga in the United States.

Although most Americans take up the practice of yoga at local studios, gyms, or YMCAs, numerous questions arise in the minds of beginners that they find difficult to ask yoga teachers in the class setting. Yoga students are generally looking for a meditative movement practice, hoping to reduce stress, increase flexibility and strength, and improve overall physical fitness. However, besides the practice on the mat, students have numerous questions on the benefits and risks of yoga poses, how to develop a personal practice, what to practice and when, how to integrate yoga into their daily lives, and the historical origins and philosophical background of yoga. This book will attempt to address some common questions students may have at the outset of developing a daily yoga practice.

Guide to Health Literacy

On her 13th birthday, Samantha was diagnosed with type 2 diabetes. She consulted her mom and her aunt, both of whom also have type 2 diabetes, and decided to go with their strategy of managing diabetes by taking insulin. As a result of participating in an after-school program at her middle school that focused on health literacy, she learned that she can help manage the level of glucose in her bloodstream by counting her carbohydrate intake, following a diabetic diet, and exercising regularly. But, what exactly should she do? How does she keep track of her carbohydrate intake? What is a diabetic diet? How long should she exercise and what type of exercise should she do? Samantha is a visual learner, so she turned to her favorite source of media, YouTube, to answer these questions. She found videos from individuals around the world sharing their experiences and tips, doctors (or at least people who have "Dr." in their YouTube channel names), government agencies such as the National Institutes of Health, and even video clips from cat lovers who have cats with diabetes. With guidance from the librarian and the health and science teachers at her school, she assessed the credibility of the information in these videos and even compared their suggestions to some of the print resources that she was able to find at her school library. Now, she knows exactly how to count her carbohydrate level, how to prepare and follow a diabetic diet, and how much (and what) exercise is needed daily. She intends to share her findings with her mom and her aunt, and now she wants to create a chart that summarizes what she has learned that she can share with her doctor.

Samantha's experience is not unique. She represents a shift in our society; an individual no longer views himself or herself as a passive recipient of medical care but as an active mediator of his or her own health. However, in this era when any individual can post his or her opinions and experiences with a particular health condition online with just a few clicks or publish a memoir, it is vital that people know how to assess the credibility of health information. Gone are the days when "publishing" health information required intense vetting. The health information landscape is highly saturated, and people have innumerable sources where they can find information about practically any health topic. The sources (whether print, online, or a person) that an individual consults for health information are crucial because the accuracy and trustworthiness of the information can potentially affect his or her overall health. The ability to find, select, assess, and use health information constitutes a type of literacy—health literacy—that everyone must possess.

THE DEFINITION AND PHASES OF HEALTH LITERACY

One of the most popular definitions for health literacy comes from Ratzan and Parker (2000), who describe health literacy as "the degree to which individuals have the capacity to obtain, process, and understand basic health information and services needed to make appropriate health decisions." Recent research has extrapolated health literacy into health literacy bits, further shedding light on the multiple phases and literacy practices that are embedded within the multifaceted concept of health literacy. Although this research has focused primarily on online health information seeking, these health literacy bits are needed to successfully navigate both print and online sources. There are six phases of health information seeking: (1) Information Need Identification and Question Formulation, (2) Information Search, (3) Information Comprehension, (4) Information Assessment, (5) Information Management, and (6) Information Use.

The first phase is the *information need identification and question formulation phase*. In this phase, one needs to be able to develop and refine a range of questions to frame one's search and understand relevant health terms. In the second phase, *information search*, one has to possess appropriate searching skills, such as using proper keywords and correct spelling in search terms, especially when using search engines and databases. It is also crucial to understand how search engines work (i.e., how search results are derived, what the order of the search results means, how to use the snippets that are provided in the search results list to select websites, and how to determine which listings are ads on a search engine results page). One also has to limit reliance on surface characteristics, such as the design of a website or a book (a website or book that appears to have a lot of information or looks aesthetically pleasant does not necessarily mean it has good information) and language used (a website or book that utilizes jargon, the keywords that one used to conduct the search, or the word "information" does not necessarily indicate it will have good information). The next phase is *information comprehension*, whereby one needs to have the ability to read, comprehend, and recall the information (including textual, numerical, and visual content) one has located from the books and/or online resources.

To assess the credibility of health information (*information assessment* phase), one needs to be able to evaluate information for accuracy, evaluate how current the information is (e.g., when a website was last updated or when a book was published), and evaluate the creators of the source—for example, examine site sponsors or type of sites (.com, .gov, .edu, or .org) or the author of a book (practicing doctor, a celebrity doctor, a patient of a specific disease, etc.) to determine the believability of the person/organization providing the information. Such credibility perceptions tend to become generalized, so they must be frequently reexamined (e.g., the belief that a specific news agency always has credible health information needs continuous vetting). One also needs to evaluate the credibility of the medium (e.g., television, Internet, radio, social media, and book) and evaluate—not just accept without questioning—others' claims regarding the validity of a site, book, or other specific source of information. At this stage, one has to "make sense of information gathered from diverse sources by identifying misconceptions, main and supporting ideas, conflicting information, point of view, and biases" (American Association of School Librarians [AASL], 2009, p. 13) and conclude which sources/information are valid and accurate by using conscious strategies rather than simply using intuitive judgments or "rules of thumb." This phase is the most challenging segment of health information seeking and serves as a determinant of success (or lack thereof) in the information-seeking process. The following section on Sources of Health Information further explains this phase.

The fifth phase is *information management*, whereby one has to organize information that has been gathered in some manner to ensure easy retrieval and use in the future. The last phase is *information use*, in which one will synthesize information found across various resources, draw conclusions, and locate the answer to his or her original question and/ or the content that fulfills the information need. This phase also often involves implementation, such as using the information to solve a health problem; make health-related decisions; identify and engage in behaviors that will help a person to avoid health risks; share the health information found with family members and friends who may benefit from it; and advocate more broadly for personal, family, or community health.

THE IMPORTANCE OF HEALTH LITERACY

The conception of health has moved from a passive view (someone is either well or ill) to one that is more active and process based (someone is working toward preventing or managing disease). Hence, the dominant focus has shifted from doctors and treatments to patients and prevention, resulting in the need to strengthen our ability and confidence (as patients and consumers of health care) to look for, assess, understand, manage, share, adapt, and use health-related information. An individual's health literacy level has been found to predict his or her health status better than age, race, educational attainment, employment status, and income level (National Network of Libraries of Medicine, 2013). Greater health literacy also enables individuals to better communicate with health care providers such as doctors, nutritionists, and therapists, as they can pose more relevant, informed, and useful questions to health care providers. Another added advantage of greater health literacy is better information-seeking skills, not only for health but also in other domains, such as completing assignments for school.

SOURCES OF HEALTH INFORMATION: THE GOOD, THE BAD, AND THE IN-BETWEEN

For generations, doctors, nurses, nutritionists, health coaches, and other health professionals have been the trusted sources of health information. Additionally, researchers have found that young adults, when they have health-related questions, typically turn to a family member who has had firsthand experience with a health condition because of their family member's close proximity and because of their past experience with, and trust in, this individual. Expertise should be a core consideration when consulting a person, website, or book for health information. The credentials and background of the person or author and conflicting interests of the author (and his or her organization) must be checked and validated to ensure the likely credibility of the health information they are conveying. While books often have implied credibility because of the peer-review process involved, self-publishing has challenged this credibility, so qualifications of book authors should also be verified. When it comes to health information, currency of the source must also be examined. When examining health information/studies presented, pay attention to the exhaustiveness of research methods utilized to offer recommendations or conclusions. Small and nondiverse sample size is often—but not always—an indication of reduced credibility. Studies that confuse correlation with causation is another potential issue to watch for. Information seekers must also pay attention to the sponsors of the research studies. For example, if a study is sponsored by manufacturers of drug Y and the study recommends that drug Y is the best treatment to manage or cure a disease, this may indicate a lack of objectivity on the part of the researchers.

The Internet is rapidly becoming one of the main sources of health information. Online forums, news agencies, personal blogs, social media sites, pharmacy sites, and celebrity "doctors" are all offering medical and health information targeted to various types of people in regard to all types of diseases and symptoms. There are professional journalists, citizen journalists, hoaxers, and people paid to write fake health news on various sites that may appear to have a legitimate domain name and may even have authors who claim to have professional credentials, such as an MD. All these sites *may* offer useful information or information that appears to be useful and relevant; however, much of the information may be debatable and may fall into gray areas that require readers to discern credibility, reliability, and biases.

While broad recognition and acceptance of certain media, institutions, and people often serve as the most popular determining factors to assess credibility of health information among young people, keep in mind that there are legitimate Internet sites, databases, and books that publish health information and serve as sources of health information for doctors, other health sites, and members of the public. For example, MedlinePlus (https://medlineplus.gov) has trusted sources on over 975 diseases and conditions and presents the information in easy-to-understand language.

The chart here presents factors to consider when assessing credibility of health information. However, keep in mind that these factors function only as a guide and require continuous updating to keep abreast with the changes in the landscape of health information, information sources, and technologies.

The chart can serve as a guide; however, approaching a librarian about how one can go about assessing the credibility of both print and online health information is far more effective than using generic checklist-type

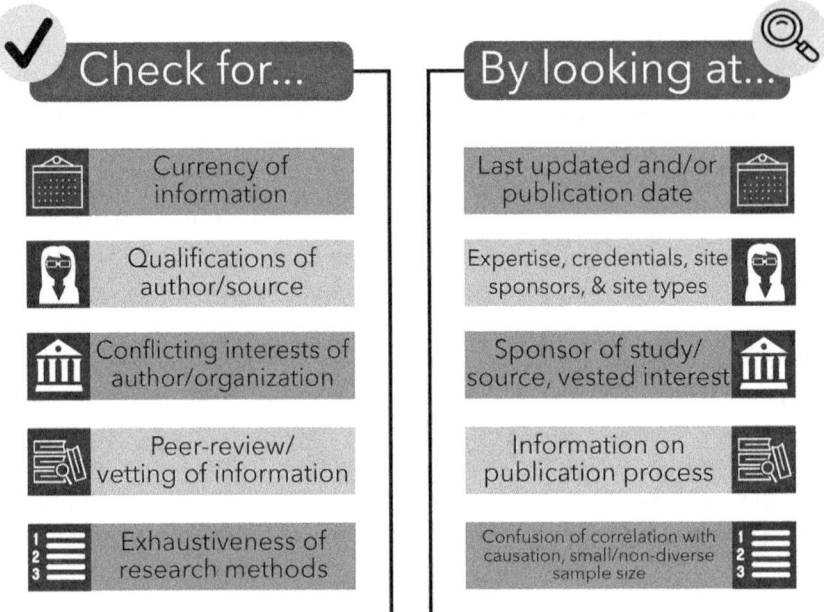

All images from flaticon.com

tools. While librarians are not health experts, they can apply and teach patrons strategies to determine the credibility of health information.

With the prevalence of fake sites and fake resources that appear to be legitimate, it is important to use the following health information assessment tips to verify health information that one has obtained (St. Jean et al., 2015, p. 151):

- **Don't assume you are right**: Even when you feel very sure about an answer, keep in mind that the answer may not be correct, and it is important to conduct (further) searches to validate the information.
- **Don't assume you are wrong**: You may actually have correct information, even if the information you encounter does not match—that is, you may be right and the resources that you have found may contain false information.
- **Take an open approach**: Maintain a critical stance by not including your preexisting beliefs as keywords (or letting them influence your choice of keywords) in a search, as this may influence what it is possible to find out.
- **Verify, verify, and verify**: Information found, especially on the Internet, needs to be validated, no matter how the information appears on

the site (i.e., regardless of the appearance of the site or the quantity of information that is included).

Health literacy comes with experience navigating health information. Professional sources of health information, such as doctors, health care providers, and health databases, are still the best, but one also has the power to search for health information and then verify it by consulting with these trusted sources and by using the health information assessment tips and guide shared previously.

Mega Subramaniam, PhD
Associate Professor, College of Information
Studies, University of Maryland

REFERENCES AND FURTHER READING

American Association of School Librarians (AASL). (2009). *Standards for the 21st-century learner in action.* Chicago, IL: American Association of School Librarians.

Hilligoss, B., & Rieh, S.-Y. (2008). Developing a unifying framework of credibility assessment: Construct, heuristics, and interaction in context. *Information Processing & Management, 44*(4), 1467–1484.

Kuhlthau, C. C. (1988). Developing a model of the library search process: Cognitive and affective aspects. *Reference Quarterly, 28*(2), 232–242.

National Network of Libraries of Medicine (NNLM). (2013). Health literacy. Bethesda, MD: National Network of Libraries of Medicine. Retrieved from nnlm.gov/outreach/consumer/hlthlit.html

Ratzan, S. C., & Parker, R. M. (2000). Introduction. In C. R. Selden, M. Zorn, S. C. Ratzan, & R. M. Parker (Eds.), *National Library of Medicine current bibliographies in medicine: Health literacy.* NLM Pub. No. CBM 2000–1. Bethesda, MD: National Institutes of Health, U.S. Department of Health and Human Services.

St. Jean, B., Taylor, N. G., Kodama, C., & Subramaniam, M. (February 2017). Assessing the health information source perceptions of tweens using card-sorting exercises. *Journal of Information Science.* Retrieved from http://journals.sagepub.com/doi/abs/10.1177/0165551516687728

St. Jean, B., Subramaniam, M., Taylor, N. G., Follman, R., Kodama, C., & Casciotti, D. (2015). The influence of positive hypothesis testing on youths' online health-related information seeking. *New Library World, 116*(3/4), 136–154.

Subramaniam, M., St. Jean, B., Taylor, N. G., Kodama, C., Follman, R., & Casciotti, D. (2015). Bit by bit: Using design-based research to improve the health literacy of adolescents. *JMIR Research Protocols*, 4(2), paper e62. Retrieved from http://www.ncbi.nlm.nih.gov/pmc /articles/PMC4464334/

Valenza, J. (2016, November 26). Truth, truthiness, and triangulation: A news literacy toolkit for a "post-truth" world [Web log]. Retrieved from http://blogs.slj.com/neverendingsearch/2016/11/26/truth-truthiness-tri angulation-and-the-librarian-way-a-news-literacy-toolkit-for-a-post -truth-world/

Common Misconceptions about Yoga

1. YOGA CONFLICTS WITH MY RELIGION

The sense in which "religion" is used in the statement above is as per its definition, "the service and worship of God or the supernatural" (Merriam Webster dictionary) and not as in its alternative meaning of simply "a strong belief." The ancient texts on yoga philosophy mention Om, the expression of God. If the ancient yoga texts are accepted as a belief, yoga can be interpreted as a religion. However, unlike formal religions, the study and practice of yoga do not demand or require belief. Yoga is based on a firsthand experience of one's own body and mind. It involves close observation, self-study, analysis of one's body and mind, and the incremental progress toward harmony. In this approach, yoga is a science. For more information on the relation between yoga and religion, refer to Question 2.

2. THE GOAL OF YOGA IS PHYSICAL FITNESS

Increasing physical strength and gaining flexibility through the practice of yoga poses (asanas) is what attracts many students to the practice of yoga. It is perfectly fine to practice yoga with the sole aim of physical fitness. However, the practice of yoga can promote more than physical well-being. Traditionally, yoga aims to still the restlessness of the mind. Yoga comprises eight interrelated and overlapping phases, the third of which is the acquiring of physical fitness through the practice of yoga poses. Physical fitness, according to yoga, is an intermediate step toward the goal of knowing oneself. Physical strength and flexibility allow the body to withstand the rigors of being still enough to observe minutely, focus acutely, and direct one's breath and mind toward the study of the true self. For more information on the application of yoga to improve physical fitness, refer to Questions 8 and 13 through 20.

3. IT TAKES LONG, STRENUOUS HOURS OF PRACTICE TO SEE THE BENEFITS OF YOGA

Whereas ancient texts on yoga direct the aspirant toward steady, prolonged, and regular practice, they also mention that the degree to which one makes progress on the path of yoga and reaps the benefits is directly proportional to the intensity one devotes to practice. This suggests that although long, hard practice may increase the magnitude of benefits if the practice is done with great intensity, even practices that are short, irregular, or do not involve intense rigor and dedication also reap some benefit. As a beginner you might need to expend more effort than when you have mastered the basics of the yoga poses. Alert observation will help you find the balance between effort and ease. Overexertion can be as counterproductive as being lackluster and inattentive in one's practice. Ancient texts such as the *Yoga Sutras* of Patanjali claim that prolonged, uninterrupted, intense practice of yoga can result in the manifestations of certain effects or powers (Sanskrit: vibhuti) in the dedicated practitioner. These include knowledge of past and present, the ability to read people's minds, the ability to become invisible, and even the ability to defy gravity and levitate. There is no recorded evidence, however, that modern practitioners have achieved any such powers. For more information on the developing of a personal yoga practice, refer to Questions 9, 31, and 36.

4. YOGA IS DANGEROUS; IT INVOLVES STANDING ON YOUR HEAD AND TWISTING INTO A PRETZEL

The practice of yoga is dangerous only if not done properly. That is why a student should search for an experienced yoga teacher and study under his or her direct supervision. This allows the beginner to start in a methodical manner, gradually developing strength, flexibility, and coordination. The practice of yoga does involve inversions and twists of the body. However, these require physical skills that are developed through prolonged, dedicated practice and are not to be attempted in the initial stages. All traditions of yoga have systematized ways of introducing new students to the practice of yoga that have been refined over time, thereby reducing the probability of injury while mindfully pushing the limits of the student's capacity. Even seemingly simple practices like breath control (Pranayama) can be fraught with dangers if not practiced properly, preferably under the guidance of an able teacher. You can avoid injury during your practice of yoga by adopting the right attitude and approach to yoga. This means that you should not approach yoga with an intense, single-minded goal to accomplishing difficult asanas. Your practice of yoga should be more about developing a deep, sustainable relationship with your body, mind, and spirit than about increasing your repertoire of difficult poses. Yoga is based on a philosophy of ahiṃsa (nonviolence), abhyasa (dedicated practice), and vairagya (detachment from the results of your actions). In your practice, it is important to not mentally or physically overdo your effort, as that is akin to being violent toward yourself. Practicing yoga with a basic knowledge of the underlying philosophy prevents injuries that arise from a result-oriented, competitive, and overzealous approach to life that may be ingrained in us through social conditioning. For more information on the risks and concerns regarding yoga practice, refer to Questions 21 to 31.

5. YOGA IS A NEW AGE FAD

Yoga developed in the northern Indian Indus-Saraswati civilization about 5,000 years ago. The word "yoga," meaning union or addition, is first found in the ancient Indian text called the *Rig Veda*, a collection of Hindu hymns in Sanskrit. Historians date this text between 1700 and 1100 BCE. The first detailed written treatise of yoga is the *Yoga Sutras* by Patanjali, written around 400 CE. Although currently the most popular text on yoga, the *Yoga Sutras* is a compilation from even older traditions. Thus, we see that the modern-day practice of yoga stems from ancient traditions and is not a New Age fad. Even in the distant past, yoga is believed to have spread to Africa and Europe through the work of monks, merchants, teachers, and migrants who traveled from India to distant parts of the world. In recent history, the yoga teacher who promoted a deep curiosity for yoga in the West was Swami Vivekananda, who traveled from Kolkata, India, to Chicago in 1894 to attend the Parliament of Religions. Since then, numerous yoga teachers have spread the practice throughout the United States. For more information about the ancient lineages of yoga, refer to Questions 1 to 6.

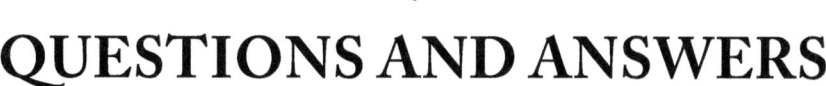

QUESTIONS AND ANSWERS

❖❖ General Information

1. What is yoga?

So vast and expansive is the subject of yoga that even lifelong students and teachers of yoga find it difficult to define it succinctly. Yoga is a comprehensive, continuously evolving system of improving the all-around well-being of human beings at all stages of their lives and abilities with the expressed aim of attaining optimum physical and mental health and a state of union with everything in the cosmos. This would be an inclusive definition for yoga, although a perfect definition would be challenging and is currently the subject of intense academic and philosophical study.

An important point to note is that although in the West yoga is often equated with a series of physical postures and breathing techniques, it is not entirely true. Physical postures or "asanas" constitute the third limb of the eightfold path of yoga. The purpose of these rigorous asanas is to equip the body with the strength and fortitude that is needed to sit still for prolonged periods of meditation. Physical postures, or asanas, in the context of yoga are not an end in themselves. Pranayamas, often translated as breathing techniques, constitute the fourth limb in the eightfold path of yoga. In Sanskrit, Pranayama is a composite word consisting of "prana" meaning life force and "ayama" meaning extension. Pranayama essentially uses the breath as a tool as breathing is the only biological process that can either be completely automatic or be performed either under total voluntary control. Pranayama is also used as a technique to develop concentration and extend the awareness of our life force. The practices of asana and pranayama are aimed at attaining a state of yoga or union. Note that in this sense, yoga is not the preparatory step for developing a connection with everything around you but rather the state of complete connectivity itself.

Perhaps the most succinct definition of yoga is present in the writings of Patanjali. Patanjali states in the second verse of the *Yoga Sutras*: "Yogas citta-vrtti-nirodhah," which is translated as "Yoga is the stilling of the changing states of the mind." This definition, similar to definitions from various other overlapping traditions of ancient India, zeroes in on the point that yoga is a practice that allows an individual to control his or her own mental tendencies through the stepping stool of rigorous physical control mastered through asanas or postures, followed by control of the breath, with the ultimate aim of gaining freedom from the suffering that having a body entails. For example, in the *Katha Upanishad*, another ancient Indian philosophical text, yoga is defined as the state attained when the sense organs are within one's control. *The Bhagavad Gita*, one of the most popular texts of yoga, defines yoga as "evenness of the mind" understood as a mind that does not become depressed in the face of adversities or ecstatic in the face of joy but is even and unruffled under all conditions.

For the beginner not inclined to delve into philosophical and metaphysical studies just yet, yoga offers a step-by-step path to self-discovery that has been refined and perfected over eons. In an age overwrought by sensory stimulation in a myriad forms, yoga provides a substantial and effective tool with which the body can be strengthened and calmed while gaining greater control of our perceptions by drawing and directing our senses inward, thereby preventing us from being a slave to external stimuli and our instinctive nature.

Incidentally, words related to "yoga" that you might come across are "yogi" or "yogin." "Yogi" and "yogin" or "yogini" indicate individuals who practice yoga—traditionally serious practitioners of yoga who have dedicated their lives to the physical and spiritual practice of yoga. "Yogi" denotes the masculine form whereas "yogin" or "yogini" is the feminine form.

2. Is yoga a religion? Do I have to follow a certain religion to do yoga?

Although yoga develops from an ancient Hindu spiritual practice, one need not be religious or adopt any religion for that matter to benefit from the practice of yoga. Yoga; its benefits on the body, mind, and spirit; and its intellectual understanding are based on direct firsthand experience and not only on ancient religious texts, however erudite or profound.

The current discipline and knowledge of yoga stems from ancient spiritual practices and studies. Although these spiritual practices are now considered the religion of Hinduism, yoga itself is not a religion. This is primarily because the practice of yoga does not require the practitioner to be part of any religious system or even believe in God or any supernatural force or accept anything based on blind faith. A practitioner of yoga can—and, according to the ancient texts, even should—study yoga and benefit from it based on his or her own personal experiences, building up the practice as physical and mental capacities increase. In this sense, yoga is not a religion or a philosophy but rather firsthand, evidence-based, methodical knowledge that can be equated to a science.

Yoga texts emphasize the central need for self-study (Svadyaya) and questioning everything as part of the practice. Yoga is not dependent on faith. A student, whether an atheist, agnostic, or believer in any form of faith, is usually drawn to the practice of yoga due to the firsthand evidence of increased well-being that the practice fosters. This itself is in direct contrast to any ritualized religious practice that is based on blind faith and conformation to dogmatic doctrines.

Yoga encourages the development of powers of discriminating between the real and unreal. This power of discrimination between the real and unreal, according to yoga, develops through listening (shravana), reflection (manana), and becoming one with the truth (niddhyasana). These discourses on the development of the powers of keen observation of one's own self and surroundings, reflection on what one has directly observed, and the realization of the ultimate truth through critical questioning constitute a systematic path far removed from faith and religion.

Interestingly, authorities, teachers, and practitioners, particularly in the West, differ in their opinions on whether yoga is to be considered a pure exercise or a spiritual path. In 2012, the teaching of yoga was regulated exempt from sales taxes by the New York state on the grounds that it is not "true exercise," whereas in the District of Columbia, yoga classes were subject to local taxes on the grounds that the intention with which students attend yoga classes is physical exercise. In Islamic countries like Saudi Arabia and Malaysia, the practice of yoga is permitted as long as it does not involve chanting or meditation.

Although yoga is not a religion, it involves the study of the nature of all religions, just as linguistics is not the study of any particular language but the study of the structure of all languages. Yoga transcends the segregation of knowledge and paths that investigate reality into artificial compartments such as the sciences, arts, and religion, while including aspects of all.

3. What do some of the Sanskrit words used in yoga class mean, like "Namaste" and "Om/Aum"? Is it necessary for me to remember the names of poses?

Many yoga teachers might use Sanskrit names for poses and other Sanskrit words to explain how certain poses came to be or the concept and philosophy underlying certain practices. It is not essential that you know these Sanskrit words to benefit from the practice of yoga. However, when undertaking the study of yoga, knowing the meaning of some Sanskrit words can help us make sense of, say, why certain poses are named after animals or mythological characters.

In addition, sound has a central place in the practice of yoga. In fact, there are forms of yoga based solely on sound (Naada yoga). For example, Transcendental Meditation, a form of meditation popularized by Maharshi Mahesh Yogi, is based on the regular repetitions of sounds or Sanskrit phrases. Although you may not know the Sanskrit words your teacher uses in yoga class at the beginning, pay close attention to how they are enunciated. According to the metaphysics of Naada yoga, the frequency and pattern of enunciation of Sanskrit words and phrases can affect specific energetic centers or chakras, resulting in profound changes in the body and the mind.

"Namaste" (nah-mas-stay) is usually said with a slight bow of the head toward the chest and folded hands, the entire surface of the right hand lying flat on the left and held upright in front of the chest with the fingertips aligned upward. The position of the hand, or "mudra," as it is known in Sanskrit, is called Pranam or Namaskar mudra. "Namaste" or "namaskar" is verbally uttered along with the gesture as a form of respectful greeting, both at the beginning and at the end of a meeting. In Sanskrit, it etymologically means, "I bow to you." Namah or namas means "to bow" and "te" means "you." In more elaborate definitions, it is used to convey that "the divine light in me bows to the divine light within you," "I honor you," "my soul recognizes your soul," or "we are one and the same."

Tantric philosophy teaches that the universal consciousness seeks to experience and express itself in diverse forms. It is the nature of individual forms of consciousness, such as human beings to forget this truth. According to Tantric philosophy, suffering results from the illusion of separateness and forgetting the universal oneness. Yoga and spiritual practices help to remind us of this oneness that is in our nature to forget.

Beyond a simple greeting, namaste reaffirms that beneath the outer sheaths of existence that may appear radically different, we are all one. We are made of the same life force, and we are more same than we are different.

As namaste is a greeting, it is expected that when someone greets you saying "Namaste," you respond. One can respond with "Namaste," conveying a mutual feeling of respect. Elders generally respond to younger people's greeting of "Namaste" with "Sukhino bhava," or "May you be happy."

Aum, according to Hindu philosophy, is the primordial sound that symbolizes everything that exists. Although chanting "Aum" is part of the Hindu, Buddhist, and Jain traditions, it can be chanted by anyone irrespective of religious beliefs. Its chanting resonates at the frequency of 432 Hz and is believed to be the same as the frequency of vibrations detected by sophisticated instruments in interstellar space. In Sanskrit the symbol is called Pranava, meaning "to sound out loudly," or Omkara, simply meaning "the symbol Om." The pictorial representation of the Om symbol looks like a numeral 3 with a small cursive "s" arising from its indent at the center of the digit, a "u" floating on top of this cursive "s" to the top right of the 3, with a dot on top of the "u."

In addition to greetings, chants, and mantras, usually at the beginning and end of the yoga class, you may also often hear the teacher using Sanskrit terms for the names of the different poses. Although there are English translations available for the names of yoga poses, there are several advantages to familiarizing yourself with the Sanskrit names. One of the advantages is that Sanskrit is a very precise and methodical language. As such, you'll find that the names of different poses are combinations of two or more smaller words. Therefore, once you are familiar with the root words, it is often possible to gauge what the name of a particular posture might be. For example, most yoga postures end in the word "-asana," which roughly translates as "seat." However, in Sanskrit, asana means more than simply "seated." Asana implies being seated in a calm, firm, relaxed, and poised manner with gravitas, and it has a quality of having been invited to sit in the first place. These are some nuances of the term that are lost in translation.

The reason most yoga postures end in the suffix -asana is likely that the yoga postures first described in the ancient texts were meant to allow yogis to sit for prolonged periods for purposes of study or meditation. Even as yoga developed over time to include standing poses, forward bends, backbends, inversions, and twists, the goal of these various poses has remained to develop the physical capacity to sit calmly and without discomfort so that the yogi can engage in meditative practices. Although this may seem counterintuitive—as we might think that sitting is easy—any person who attempts to sit still and focused for a prolonged period will realize the difficulties in this seemingly simple task.

"Guru" is another Sanskrit word that you might come across in yoga classes and books. Although now commonly used in the English language to mean an expert in any field, often with a twinge of sarcasm, "guru" in Sanskrit refers to a spiritual teacher held in high esteem.

Various yoga asanas, you'll find, have common prefixes and suffixes. For example, "pada" in Sanskrit means "foot" or "leg" and is found in the names of various yoga asanas, such as Prasarita Padasana (extended wide-legged posture), Padangushtasana (big toe pose), Uttana Padasana (intense stretch of the legs pose), and so on. Similarly, "hasta," meaning "hand" or "arm" in Sanskrit, is found in Padahastasana (hand to feet pose), Urdhva Hastasana (upward arm pose), Eka Hasta Bhujasana (leg over shoulder pose), and so forth. "Parshva," meaning "sideways" in Sanskrit, is seen in Parsvottanana (intense side stretch pose), Utthita Parshva Konasana (extended side angle pose), and so on. Parivritta is generally translated as "revolved" although it inherently means "to turn around." You'll find "parivritta" used in the names of yoga asanas such as Parivritta Parshva konasana (revolved side angle pose) or Parivritta Trikonasana (revolved triangle pose). "Urdhva" in Sanskrit means "upward" and is found in the name of yoga poses such as Urdhvahastasana (upward arm pose), Urdhva Mukha Shvanasana (upward facing dog pose), or Urdhva Dhanurasana (upward bow pose). On the other hand the prefix "Adho" in Sanskrit signifies "downward," and you'll find it in the names of common poses such as Adho Mukha Shvanasana (downward facing dog pose), Adho Mukha Virasana (downward facing hero pose), or Adho Mukha Dandasana (downward facing staff pose, also known as plank pose). "Baddha" in Sanskrit means "bound," and it is commonly used in the name of yoga asanas that involve clasping the arms together or bring the limbs close and holding them together, such as Baddha Konasana (bound angle pose) or Baddha Virabhadrasana (bound warrior or humble warrior pose). Another common pair of words often used in the names of yogasanas are "paschima" and "purva." Although these words literally mean "west" and "east," respectively, in the context of yoga, east refers to the front of the body and the west refers to the back of the body, perhaps because yoga has long been practiced early in the morning, facing the sun, which places the front of the body to the east. These directional prefixes are generally used in the names of yogasanas such as Paschimottanasana (intense stretch of the back of the body), Paschima Namaskarasana (greeting the west or greeting the back of the body), or Purvottanasana (intense stretch of the front of the body).

In the beginning, it might feel overwhelming when the teacher uses Sanskrit names in class, either by themselves or together with English names, and experienced students immediately know what poses to get into! Don't sweat if you cannot remember the names. A good yoga teacher will be aware of new students in the class and guide you accordingly, either by demonstrating each new pose or using another student as a model. If you find yourself getting curious about what the names of poses mean, you can always look them up on the internet. Some interesting books on the origin of the names of yoga poses are listed in the bibliography at the end of this book.

4. What is pranayama?

Pranayama, an integral element in the yogic discipline, is the fourth limb in the eightfold path of ashtanga yoga. Although popularly recognized as a set of calming breathing exercises, pranayama aims to use the breath as a tool to gain access to the movements of the mind and the constant distractions in our awareness and consciousness. "Prana" refers to the breath, energetic source, or life force. "Yama" refers to restraint, control, or consolidation. Patanajali's *Yoga Sutras* state that the aim of the practice of pranayama is to make the breath long, deep, and silent. The practice of pranayama energizes the body and trains the mind for the next stages of yoga—dharana (concentration), dhyana (meditation), and samadhi (self-realization).

A variety of breathing techniques, both calming and invigorating, are used to this end. For example, several levels of Ujjayi, or the "breath of victory," involves long, uninterrupted inhalations or exhalations or both while constricting the glottis at the back of the mouth to produce a gentle sound much like the sound of the ocean from a distance. The Ujjayi breath has a calming or invigorating effect depending on whether the exhalation or inhalation is extended, respectively. Bhramari is another pranayama that is accompanied by a hum like the sound of bees, emanating from the base of the throat on the exhalation and ushers in a deep sense of calm and relaxation. Kapalabhati pranayama, popularly known as the breath of fire, literally means "skull perception" ("kapala" meaning skull and "bhati" meaning perception or knowledge). Kapalabhati involves strong bursts of short exhalations accompanied by the contraction and recoiling of the lower abdomen between the naval and the pubis, followed by long, passive inhalations. This pranayama is practiced as a cleansing technique or kriya and has a long list of benefits. Some of the benefits of Kapalabhati include relief of sinus-related issues, increased blood circulation, and increased metabolism.

Pranayama is a subtle practice that requires the preparation of the body and mind though asana, or physical postures, first. In many traditional schools of yoga, pranayama is only taught to students once they have an established daily practice of asana and are well grounded in their understanding and practice of the yamas and niyamas (universal rules and observances).

Moreover, unlike asana, which can be learned, at least at a basic level, from books and other indirect media, pranayama should be learned under the guidance of a skilled teacher. This is because it is a subtle practice wherein errors in the method of practice are difficult to detect on one's own. If practiced improperly, pranayama can have serious and harmful consequences. Unlike asanas, during which an improper practice results in pain in a physical part of the body and therefore can be avoided, the detrimental consequences of pranayama are usually subtle and difficult to associate directly with the specific incorrectness in the method of practicing pranayama. For example, incorrect pranayama practice can cause restless or reduced sleep, increased irritability, migraines, elevated or low body temperatures, increased or reduced appetite, heartburn, fluctuations in blood pressure, dizziness, and a gamut of other mild to severe issues that are difficult to directly correlate with the practice of pranayama. In severe cases, practicing complex pranayama such as Kapalabhati and Bhastrika without proper guidance has been reported to cause cardiac failure. In milder cases, sometimes direct physical pain arises from pranayama as well, such as a soreness in the intercostal muscles and ribs with the repeated expanding of the ribcage during exaggerated inhalation. This can be readily corrected by easing up on the effort expended in breathing in.

In fact, one of the dangers of practicing pranayama on your own is the instinctual application of willpower in the form of excessive effort. In our day-to-day lives in school, sports, and work, emphasis lies on applying willpower to achieve goals. Even in the practice of asana, the use of some effort or willpower is necessary. However, in the practice of pranayama, setting your mind on its usual groove of accomplishing something cannot only be unproductive but also harmful. Exerting effort inevitably results in stress. Stress in the subtle art of breathing and breath control can strain the internal organs and the mind. The traditional Indian setting of learning pranayama from an experienced guru in quiet, secure surroundings over prolonged periods involved a mental attitude of surrender, dedication, and spirituality that is seldom accessible in the modern setting of a yoga class. A trained teacher, however, can guide you into the mental approach that is a prerequisite to the safe learning and practice of pranayama.

During the time we spend awake, it is usually the sympathetic nervous system that is in control. The sympathetic nervous system is that part of the autonomic nervous system that prepares the body for intense physical activity by increasing the heartrate and is responsible for such biological responses as the flight-or-fight response. Research shows some pranayama techniques such as alternate nostril breathing, where fingers are used to apply gentle pressure on the outside of each nostril sequentially to direct the breath through one nostril or the other, tone the parasympathetic nervous system and also affect electrical activity in the brain.

5. When and where did people first begin practicing yoga, and when did it come to the United States?

The earliest mention of yoga is found in the ancient philosophical texts of India, in the Indus-Saraswati civilization about 5,000 years ago. However, yoga was practiced long before it had ever been written about. This is because a large part of the transfer of knowledge from teacher to student in ancient India, happened through a process called sruti. Loosely translated as "listening," sruti involves the concentrated listening, memorization, assimilation, and reflection that students were expected to perform under the guidance of their gurus.

Early writing was performed on fragile palm leaves. So even if the early yoga practitioners and teachers had written about yoga, these writings were lost, damaged, or destroyed. The first written record of yoga is found in the Rig Veda. The Vedas are a collection of hymns and songs written by various saints and priests. The written text of the Rig Veda dates between 1700 and 1100 BCE. But even before it was written down, it was preserved in the oral traditions. Yoga developed as a spiritual practice in India before it was documented in the Rig Vedas between 1700 and 1100 BCE and was passed down through the generations as a sacred practice.

Yoga traveled outside India with traveling saints, ascetics, merchants, and householders who were yoga practitioners and traveled to different countries. The missionaries responsible for the spread of Buddhism also helped spread yoga beyond India. The spread of yoga from India to

Europe and the Americas has largely been as a physical practice, whereas its spread to the far East, including Japan and China, has occurred as a holistic spiritual practice.

The social, cultural, religious, and spiritual context of yoga practice in India has only been transmitted to the West in limited pockets of highly devoted, serious students. International socioreligious conferences such as the Parliament of the World's Religions and organizations such as the Self-Realization Fellowship have had a strong influence in bringing the practice of yoga to the West with the philosophical and cultural context in which yoga developed.

Swami Vivekananda (1863–1902) disciple of Sri Ramakrishna represented India and Hinduism at the Parliament of World Religions in Chicago in 1893 and later established the first Vedanta Society in 1894 in New York. His famous speeches were among the first to pique U.S. interest in Vedanta philosophy and the path of yoga.

Paramahansa Yogananda (1893–1952) founded the Self-Realization Fellowship, an international spiritual organization, in Los Angeles, California, in 1920. Another renowned Indian, Jiddu Krishnamurti (1895–1986), though not yoga teacher per se, spread the concepts of a meditative and discerning life through his talks and writings. Yoga has been taught as part of the school curriculum in all Krishnamurti Foundation Schools in the United States and United Kingdom since its inception in 1928, such as the Oak Grove School in Ojai, California, and the Brockwood Park School in the United Kingdom. This has been pivotal in educating generations of Western students in the holistic understanding of the practice of yoga.

Perhaps the greatest impact of spreading yoga in the West as a rigorous physical practice and beyond has been through the teachings of the students of the South Indian yoga masters Tirumalai Krishnamacharya (1888–1989), BKS Iyengar (1918–2014), K. Pattabhi Jois (1915–2009), and T. K. V. Desikachar (1938–2016). Other popular conduits of the spread of yoga in the United States has been through the Chinmaya Mission, founded by Chinmaya Saraswati in 1953, and the International Sivananda Yoga Vedanta Centers, founded by Swami Vishnudevananda in 1959.

Historically, India was invaded by the English, French, Dutch, Greek, Portuguese, Spanish, Mongols, and the Arabs, and it was colonized for hundreds of years. Together with natural resources such as food and minerals that were transmitted abroad, language, books, and people also moved as a result of these invasions. The culture and philosophy of India, including the practice of yoga, also spread because of the repeated invasions and prolonged colonization of India.

In more recent history, many U.S. thinkers disillusioned by the contemporary culture of consumerism, competition, and the various maladies in Western society traveled to India and studied yoga. They brought back to the United States not only the physical practice of asanas but also the wisdom of the ancient spiritual texts. An example of such an American yogi is Ram Dass, previously known as Dr. Richard Alpert, a Harvard psychology professor, infamous for his use of psychedelics, who later traveled to India and studied yoga. He returned to the United States to write several popular books on yoga and was pivotal in spreading the knowledge of yoga through generations of Americans.

6. What are the different types of yoga?

With the increasing popularity and spread of yoga, various styles have emerged from the traditional schools, differing largely in the kind and type of yoga asanas or postures that the style emphasizes rather than differences in the philosophical underpinnings. This is not surprising, as yoga is not a rigid or dogmatic study nor is the path patented by commercial laws. Yoga encourages individual understanding and expression. This has resulted in the development of unique styles of teaching and practicing asanas based on one's goals and capacities. Keeping this is mind, here is a brief discussion of the "types" of yoga you might encounter as you search for a class that suits you. This classification is based on two broad criteria: first, the traditional schools or paths of yoga and second, the modern forms of yoga.

Traditional schools or paths of yoga

Hatha yoga: Most forms of yoga that have become popular in the West emphasize the practice of physical postures and, to a lesser extent, various forms of breathing techniques. All such types of yoga fall under the traditional category of Hatha yoga. "Hatha" is a Sanskrit term that can be interpreted in two ways: it means "willful" or "effortful." In this sense the practice of yoga wherein effort is needed and is central to the practice can be called Hatha yoga. In a different interpretation, Hatha is a combined word composed of "Ha," meaning "the sun," and "tha" meaning "the moon." In this sense Hatha yoga is understood as the practice that infuses us with balance, bringing into equilibrium the opposing elements in our selves. True to the traditional sense, Hatha yoga prepares the body and mind for Dhyana, or meditation, by aligning and strengthening the body for the stillness that is required for meditation. The Hatha Yoga Pradipika, written by Svatmarama in the fifteenth century, gives detailed descriptions of yoga asanas. However, this authoritative text, too, like Patanjali's *Yoga Sutras*, is a compilation based on knowledge that was handed down through generations (sruti) and is not an original composition.

Bhakti yoga: Bhakti yoga is one of the four major paths of yoga as discussed in the ancient texts of the Vedantas: Bhakti yoga, Gyana yoga, Karma yoga, and Raja yoga. "Bhakti" is a Sanskrit term translated as "an intense love for God." Bhakti yoga is not a sequence of postures but is rather a philosophy and a way of life that consciously infuses every action with love for the divine. Writers on Bhakti yoga mention it not only as a complement to Ashtanga yoga but also as an alternative path in its own right to achieve the goal of yoga, or "union with all." Bhakti, often explained as "love for love's sake," is believed to be greater than Karma yoga, or the "yoga of action and doing," because unlike action, which progresses toward a goal, love is a goal in itself.

Karma yoga: Karma yoga is yoga in action. It is the path of focused, dedicated work, whatever the choice of work might be. Karma yoga, as the Bhagavad Gita expounds, is letting go of the thought of any specific goal, whether desirable goals in the form of victory or undesirable goals in the form of failure, and immersing oneself wholly in the action at hand. Instead of considering it a separate practice, Karma yoga can be practiced regardless of one's professional or spiritual path.

Gyana yoga: Gyana yoga is believed to be the most difficult of the four paths of yoga. Gyana is the path of knowledge and wisdom to attain the state of union with all. It involves the careful discrimination between the real and the unreal through the use of reason and logic. The path of Gyana yoga involves studying spiritual texts; questioning what one studies in texts and sees in one's surroundings; and using one's intellect to listen, reflect, and meditate. The reason the journey to liberation through Gyana yoga is considered more difficult than others is that it is easy to be swayed by one's intellectual attainments, resulting in an inflation of the ego, which is an impediment on the yogic path. Therefore, cultivating humility and compassion helps maintain balance along the path of Gyana yoga.

Raja yoga: Raja yoga, or the "royal path," is the path of meditation, mantras, and skill in action. Essentially identical to Ashtanga yoga, Raja yoga seeks to unify the body and mind. Raja yoga relies on direct perception and does not require the adoption of any faith or religious belief system. Through the practice of balance in one's daily lifestyle and taking complete responsibility for one's own thoughts and actions, the Raja yogi seeks liberation.

Kundalini yoga: Kundalini is a traditional blend of Bhakti yoga and Raja yoga that stems from the Hindu concept that the infinite potential dormant in the individual self lies in a tight coil at the base of the spine. In Sanskrit the term for "coil" is "kundali." Kundalini is often likened to a coiled snake at the base of the spine. The various physical and spiritual practices in Kundalini yoga are aimed at creating an energetic awareness of the spine and ultimately to awaken the seat of energy at the base of the spine.

Ashtanga Yoga: Ashtanga yoga in the traditional sense is often confused with Ashtanga Yoga as understood and practiced currently. Ashtanga yoga describes the traditional eightfold path of yoga as described in Patanjali's *Yoga Sutras*: yama, niyama, asana, pranayama, pratyahara, dhyana, and samadhi. "Ashta" means "eight," and "anga" means "limb" in Sanskrit. However, in recent times, the style of yoga consisting of six defined sequences, as taught by Sri Pattabhi K. Jois, is popularly known as Ashtanga yoga. The modern Ashtanga yoga is a defined system of sequentially arranged poses that go from beginner level sequences to advanced sequences. The sequences are repeated and memorized through practice. The breath is intricately coordinated with the movements. The practice builds core strength and tones and energizes the body. Since the practice is repetitive, students do not have to think about creating sequences of their own but simply repeat the already choreographed sequences. There are some students who enjoy the repetitive rigor and focused discipline of this format while other who prefer to focus on specific aspects of alignment or to create their own sequences find this style less appealing.

Modern schools or types

Iyengar yoga: Iyengar yoga emphasizes alignment and thoughtful awareness in practicing Patanjali's eightfold path of yoga. Although it is not a distinct yoga path, as its originator pointed out, this method receives its name from BKS Iyengar, who taught yoga widely in both the East and the West. Iyengar yoga has become popular over the last century because of innovations in the use of various props, methodical and systematic instructions, and application of therapeutic yoga, whereby individuals can progress in a step-by-step manner through the gamut of asanas and pranayama. Some students find this alignment focused style of teaching too physical and not spiritual enough.

Vinyasa yoga: Vinyasa yoga is characterized by the stringing of yoga poses, one after the other, using the breath, without returning to a foundation asana or posture such as Tadasana after each pose. Vinyasa yoga is often called flow yoga because of the use of varied creative sequences that almost appear as a choreographed dance sequence. "Vinyasa" is a Sanskrit composite word that can be translated as "to place in a special way." Vinyasa yoga embodies and explicates the notion of parinamvada, which is the idea that life is ever-changing. Pattabhi Jois's six popular Ashtanga yoga sequences are also popularly referred to as Ashtanga Vinyasa yoga. Jois's teacher, Krishnamacharya, championed Vinyasa yoga as a transformative approach using the term in a more expansive sense to define a lifestyle of minute awareness to the rhythms of relationships, work, and play, rather than simply a sequence of asanas.

Power yoga: Vinyasa flow yoga is sometimes mistaken for power yoga. "Power yoga," a term coined in the late 1980s by Beryl Bender Birch and Bryan Kest, is essentially the modification of Ashtanga yoga sequences for athletes. Power yoga aims at creating the highest levels of energy, vitality, and freedom. Generally, power yoga classes are full of intense activity, loud music, temperatures hovering close to 90 degrees Fahrenheit, and a generally amped-up, party-like atmosphere. However, the underlying intention of power yoga was to use the fitness brand to attract athletes to the deeper practice of yoga by developing an awareness of balance, strength, flexibility, and the inner self.

Yin yoga: Yin yoga, originally introduced by Paulie Zink, is characterized by holding poses for three to five minutes each. Thought of as a passive, restorative, and calming practice, Yin yoga aims to stretch the connective tissues, particularly around the major joints in the knee, pelvis, and spine. Although generally thought of as a restorative, gentle form of yoga, due to the prolonged periods that it is customary to hold poses in Yin yoga, it is also difficult for beginners, who may not have the flexibility, stamina, or endurance to hold poses for extended periods. Correct alignment and proper sequencing of poses is crucial when practicing Yin yoga as it requires an awareness of balance, strength, and endurance.

Yoga therapy: Although all yoga is essentially therapeutic, there is a clear distinction between a yoga class and a yoga therapy session. Inherently, yoga therapy addresses the specific needs of individuals such as particular joint issues, stiffness, lack of strength, sleeplessness, fatigue, pregnancy, and pain management. The yoga therapist, unlike a yoga teacher, first assesses the requirement of the client or student and then uses yoga tools, including asana, pranayama, and meditation, to address the client's specific issues. Although it is common for a student to receive therapeutic benefits in the different types of yoga classes, yoga therapy puts the specific therapeutic needs of the student or client front and center and uses yoga to address these needs. As such, the focus of yoga therapy is different from a yoga class, and the yoga therapist goes through a different education and comes with a different skill set. Individuals needing specific attention and who are comfortable with hands-on adjustments benefit from yoga therapy. For more on hands-on adjustments, see Questions 41 and 42.

Hot yoga: Hot yoga, introduced by Bikram Ghosh, is characterized by a vigorous, fixed sequence of twenty-six yoga poses practiced in a room heated from 92 to 105 degrees Fahrenheit that is maintained at a relative humidity of 40 percent. The poses involve sustained flexion and contraction of muscle groups. Performing these strenuous poses in a hot, humid room is designed to tone the muscles and increase the heart rate. Hot yoga is not advisable for individuals with heart disease, heat intolerance, and susceptibility to heat strokes.

Jivamukti yoga: Jivamukti yoga as popularly known in the United States, although based on Patanjali's Ashtanga yoga, is a branded, proprietary yoga method initiated by Sharon Gannon and David Life. It embodies the tenets of nonviolence (ahimsa), bhakti (devotion), dhyana (meditation), nada (deep listening), and shastra (spiritual study). It involves the practice of specified yoga sequences and a lifestyle of living in harmony with nature. Literally, " jivamukti" is a Sanskrit term that refers to the paths that lead to liberation or self-realization while still living.

Shivananda yoga: Shivananda yoga is a proprietary brand of yoga initiated by Swami Vishnudevananda and named after his guru Swami Shivananda. Shivananda yoga aims to develop physical, mental, and spiritual well-being through the practice of asana, pranayama, dhyana, and the study of Vedanta. Based on the Ashtanga Hatha yoga philosophy, Shivananda yoga focuses on making yoga accessible to all levels.

Aerial yoga: Aerial yoga is a recent method that involves the performance of yoga poses while suspended in a hammock. The use of the cloth hammock assists in the attainment of yoga postures that are more difficult to do on the ground and offers a supportive, exciting, and playful way to combine breath and yoga postures in a flow sequence.

Aquatic yoga: Also known as water yoga or aqua yoga, this method employs yoga principles and yoga postures to attain strength, flexibility, and balance in the environment of a warm pool. Aquatic yoga also uses props such as floaters to practice various standing yoga postures, which allows greater ease, flexibility and comfort. The buoyancy of water, in itself therapeutic, allows aquatic yoga practitioners to reduce chances of injury due to falling. However, not all hatha yoga asanas can be performed in water.

Viniyoga: "Viniyoga" is a Sanskrit term that can be translated as "use" or "application." Also based on the Ashtanga and Hatha yoga tradition and brought to the west largely through the work of the South Indian yoga master T. K. V. Desikachar and his students, Viniyoga is characterized by an emphasis of function over form in the practice of yoga postures, an emphasis on varying the breath in yoga poses to achieve different results, a balance between repetition of yoga poses and staying in a pose for prolonged periods, and unique sequencing directed toward achieving different functions.

Anusara yoga: Anusara, meaning "flowing with grace," is a multidisciplinary approach based on traditional Hatha yoga principles and nondualistic Tantric philosophy of Kashmir Shaivism. Anusara yoga is characterized by connecting and integrating an awareness of the body, mind, and spirit into the yoga poses. Classes usually begin with a philosophical discourse and chanting and work through an initial warm up and progressive sequence to a peak pose and finally wind down through a sequence of cooling down poses.

Other new and specialized forms of yoga include Acro yoga, which incorporates elements of gymnastics and acrobatics; Restorative yoga, which incorporates calming poses held for a long time and is targeted at particular muscle groups; Prenatal yoga, which focuses on poses such as hip openers to help women cope with the challenges of pregnancy and delivery; and Chair yoga, which modifies yoga poses such that they can be performed while seated on a chair and is beneficial for travelers, workers who have to sit for prolonged periods, the elderly, and the wheelchair bound. Laughing yoga, or Hasya yoga, is practice based on the belief that prolonged voluntary laughter produces the same beneficial effects as laughter that is stimulated by something humorous. Usually practiced in large groups where voluntary laughter often transforms into real laughter, this curious form of yoga has recently gained a large following globally.

7. Are there scientific or medical studies that show the efficacy of yoga?

A brief search of the authoritative and widely recognized biomedical resource Pubmed (pubmed.gov), developed and maintained by the National Library of Medicine (NLM) and National Center of the Biotechnology Information (NCBI), using the keyword "yoga" retrieves 5,551 scientific or biomedical articles on yoga as of June 22, 2020, including 960 review articles, 187 meta-analyses, 846 clinical trials, and 645 randomized controlled trials. This large number of scientific publications on yoga shows a growing interest of the biomedical community in the methods, tools, and therapeutic applications of yoga.

Scientific studies on yoga have their pros and cons. The merits include an objective insight into how yoga works, a deeper understanding of the anatomy of the human body in the context of dynamic and isometric movement, insight into how physiology can be understood and regulated internally, and the discovery of a new set of tools to understand and study the mind. The demerits are a little more difficult to see at first. One of the technical drawbacks in scientific studies on yoga is the small number of individuals these studies are conducted on (sample sizes) and the lack of randomized controls, which are key to experimental studies. Randomized controlled studies measure the effect of an intervention or practice on participants who are randomly assigned to the experimental test (in this case, a specific yoga practice), a comparable standard practice (for example, aerobics or cycling), or no test at all. At a deeper level, most of the scientific studies on yoga focus on its therapeutic aspects—how yoga can help back pain, insomnia, reduce hypertension, or increase strength and flexibility in the injured. No doubt, such studies are important and offer a valuable opportunity to develop standardized treatment protocols that can then be used in clinical and therapeutic settings. However, the drawback of zeroing in on the benefits of yoga leaves a vast arena of yoga unexplored in terms of basic scientific inquiry. This drawback can be partly attributed to the fact that the scientific method is not ideally suited to explore the subjective and intuitive realms, including even irrefutable biological facts such as the existence of consciousness.

Studies on the therapeutic benefits of yoga are numerous and growing both in quality and quantity with every passing year. For example, a recent study on patients with hypertension and type 2 diabetes shows that practicing a yoga-based meditation technique for eight weeks reduces LDL (low density lipoprotein) cholesterol levels and the gene expression levels of inflammatory proteins. Although the study included controls, the sample size of the study was small, including only twenty-one individuals who were tested after the eight-week meditation practice.

Several large-scale meta-analytical studies on yoga or research studies that statistically evaluate data from several independent studies to see overall trends have also been conducted in recent years. For example, recent meta-analytical studies show that the practice of yoga has positive effects in patients with a wide range of afflictions including fibromyalgia, Parkinson's, depression, endometriosis, a history of strokes, various kinds of pains, arthritis, and respiratory diseases.

Benefits

8. Why should I practice yoga?

Scientific research and student reviews reveal a wide array of benefits of a daily yoga practice. Both teachers and long-term practitioners strongly recommend developing a personal yoga practice at home, in addition to taking regular classes, to reap the benefits of yoga. In time, yoga increases flexibility even in individuals who feel tightness and soreness in various muscle groups.

For example, people who need to sit for long hours find that their hamstrings become tight over time. Such individuals find it particularly difficult to bend forward due to the loss of flexibility in the hamstrings. A careful, well-guided yoga practice helps stretch the hamstrings and surrounding connective tissue to increase flexibility over time. The development of strength and flexibility go hand in hand as one's yoga practice progresses. Hyperflexible people also face various challenges in the practice of yoga and must first develop the strength to prevent injuries.

In addition to providing a safe, balanced way to increase muscle strength and tone throughout the body, yoga also has several benefits on the body's subtle physiology as well as mental health. The practice of asanas, particularly pranayama, improves respiration, increases the body's energy and enthusiasm for work, and increases vitality and poise.

Some of us have a heightened metabolism while others have a sluggish metabolism. The correct sequencing of yoga poses balances the body's metabolism at the cellular level and aids hard-to-regulate functions such as digestion and the elimination of waste matter.

Although not directly targeted at weight reduction, practicing yoga regularly changes eating habits over time and burns excess reserves in the body. More importantly, a balanced practice of yoga under the guidance of a knowledgeable teacher has a profound effect on the mental balance. This effect trickles down to biological functions such as resetting our sense of fullness or satiety, giving us a sense of control over our food intake, thereby regulating body weight in the long term.

Yoga impacts all organ systems and functions in the body. But perhaps the effect is most apparent on cardiac and circulatory health. In toning and stretching the muscles, yoga also stretches the blood vessels that course through our bodies. Although some flow yoga sequences and inversions do increase heart rate, pulse rate, and blood pressure, the practice of yoga largely enhances heart and circulatory health without increasing the functional demand on the heart's activity. Yoga aims at stabilizing the breath and keeping the heart and circulatory system functioning comfortably within its normal resting limits while toning and transforming the body. Patanjali, in his Yoga Sutras, describes asanas as the balance between effort and ease. This facet of yoga, unlike any other physical practice or sport, leads to a slow, sustainable transformation of the body and mind while limiting the risk of injury.

Athletes experience improved athletic performance once they take up a regular practice of yoga. It not only recharges their mental focus but also balances the body's strength in muscles that are not commonly used in their respective sports. For example, runners and cyclists tend to have overdeveloped quadriceps, the muscles in the front of the thighs, but shortened, tight hamstrings. Practicing yoga balances the muscles on the front and back of the thighs for these athletes, giving them greater balance, flexibility, and ease of movement. Practicing yoga also protects athletes from injuries by making them more aware of their bodies and their physical and mental limits.

The muscular system is directly affected through a regular practice of yoga. Yoga builds muscle mass and tone and flushes out muscle waste such as lactic acid. Ailments directly and indirectly related to the function of muscles such as headache, backache, muscle spasms, and cramps are relieved through yoga.

In time, yoga brings greater alignment to the musculoskeletal system, increasing the energy available for activity. Bones, which we tend to think of as inert mineral structures, are in reality very much alive and require nutrition and activity for optimal health. The practice of asanas provides a balanced way of stimulating blood flow in bones, allowing different groups of bones to bear weight. Asanas internally massage the joints and fascia or connective tissue that connects bones to each other or to muscles.

Above all, yoga encourages us to systematically focus our awareness on our own body, mind, and spirit. Awareness is the first step to eliminating fear, increasing understanding, and loving yourself. Surprisingly, yoga also instills in us a sense of humor by weakening the grip of our egos on our conscious mind and helping us see the fleeting nature of physical and mental states. You will notice that many asanas in yoga involve maintaining a fine balance. This might appear to be a victory of will and determination. But a practiced yogi will say it is only possible to hold a delicate balance when you do not take yourself too seriously, when you're okay with falling out of balance and can see the funny side of it.

Through the methodical and deliberate consideration of all our limitations and talents, yoga makes us realize that all our attributes, not just balance, are in fact gifts that help us know ourselves better. And in knowing ourselves, we know the world around us. Practicing yoga teaches us why and how we must be ourselves. Yoga helps us embrace our uniqueness and love ourselves just as we are, unconditionally.

9. How can yoga help me find balance in life?

Studying and practicing yoga helps you find balance in life at several levels. We'll talk a bit about the illusive concept of balance in the context of the body, the mind, and the spirit.

You hear a lot about falling out of balance. The pressures of family and work, ambitions and expectations, and home and environment all take their toll on our bodies, even if we are not paying attention. There are certain cultures, including our own, wherein being active and working twenty-four-seven is commended. These stressful values that we absorb unconsciously as we grow up soon lead to burnout and, in severe cases, to clinical symptoms such as fatigue and depression. In Japan, they have a term for it: karoshi, which is literally translated as "overwork death."

Conscious human beings, therefore, are very intent on understanding balance and moderation and ways of achieving "work-life balance." Much of the growing interest in yoga in the West is due to its being a wonderful tool to practically understand and experience balance.

Physical balance

At the physical level, the practice of yoga asana literally teaches you the tools to align the right and left sides of body and makes you aware of your symmetry and physical tendencies, not just when you practice but also as you go about your daily life. Yoga asana teaches you how to bend forward and backward, twist, and invert, at your own pace with control from within.

Combining strengthening and stretching poses affects the nervous system. As we practice the physical asana, the focus of the mind moves inward, and we notice how the different orientations and subtle changes in alignment of the physical body alter our breath and perception.

One-legged standing poses like Vryksasana (tree pose), Virabhadrasana III (warrior pose III), Ardha Padma Uttanasana (half-lotus intense forward bend pose), Padangushtasana (hand to big toe pose) require a lot of physical and mental balance. You will learn how building and strengthening your pose from the ground up improves your sense of balance. You will learn how using different aspects of your mind, such as your imagination, can increase your feeling rootedness.

You will learn how the focused gaze of your eyes (drishti) can help you still your mind. Although the Sanskrit word "drishti" is literally translated as "sight" in English, it means more than just seeing. For example, drishti can be practiced with eyes closed, during the practice of asana or meditation to encourage a withdrawing of the senses. This promotes alignment, focus, and self-awareness. The power and importance of drishti is based on the observation that your attention is focused on the point your eyes gaze at directly and intently. Nine types of drishtis are defined in yoga, based on the point of focus. These are as follows:

> Nasagrai drishti: the nose tip (e.g., practiced in standing forward fold, Uttanasana)
> Bhrumadhye drishti: the ajna chakra, or between the eyebrows (e.g., practiced in fish pose, Matsyasana)
> Nabi chakra drishti: the navel (e.g., practiced in downward-facing dog pose, Adho Mukha Shvanasana)
> Angusthamadhye: the middle of the thumb (e.g., practiced in the fierce pose, Utkatasana)
> Hastagrai drishti: the hands (e.g., practiced in triangle pose, Trikonasana or extended side angle pose, Utthita Parshva Konasana)
> Parsva drishti: the left and the right side, considered as separate drishtis (e.g., practiced in Bharadvaja's twist pose)

Padayoragrai drishti: the toes (e.g., practiced in seated forward bend, Paschimottanasana)
Urdhva drishti: upward (e.g., practiced in warrior I, Virabhadrasana I or tree pose, Vrykshasana)

Incidentally, you will find some yoga teachers and students practice poses with their eyes closed. This is not recommended, particularly at beginner's levels. This is because drishti, or where and how you focus your eyes helps improve balance and alignment. Closing your eyes is only recommended in passive or restorative poses such as Shavasana, corpse pose, or once you have mastered balance and alignment at an expert level.

Most importantly, asana fosters a sense of noncompetitive playfulness that shows you it's okay to lose balance and fall at times and teaches you the importance of laughing at yourself and moving on. In fact, a form of yoga currently popular in India is called Laughing Yoga, in which people do simple yoga poses in large groups and take regular laughing breaks!

Mental balance

Mr. B.K.S. Iyengar said, "Yoga does not change the way we see things, it transforms the person who sees" (*Light on Life*, 2014). It is through the alignment of the body and the breath in the physical practice of yoga that you in time arrive at subtle discoveries about your intellect, your emotions and what makes you, you. Instead of talking about things as is done in say psychotherapy, yoga beings about a first-hand awareness of your own mental state in a very practical and safe way. On the very surface, you might become more aware of what relaxes you, what relieves you of your stress, and what calms you down when you're angry or sad or even exuberant. The practice of yoga sharpens your intellect and directs the focus of your mind on you. The withdrawal of the mind itself from its myriad external distractions is sufficient to increase calm. But yoga does not simply foster passive relaxation and calm; it activates mental faculties so that you gain greater control over your mental balance.

Spiritual balance

On the surface it might seem yoga is just a collection of postures requiring you to stretch and twist into a pretzel. How can such postures translate into a balanced lifestyle? Yoga is not a collection of postures. The postures you see when people talk about yoga in the media are called asana. Asanas constitute a form or stage of yoga. Yoga is a philosophy of being. It is one of the six prominent philosophies originating in ancient India.

When your physical practice of yoga reveals its mental benefits to you, you might undertake a deeper study of yoga philosophy. You will then find that asana is the third phase or stage in the eight stages of yoga. The study of the first two stages, the yamas, or ethical guidelines, and niyamas, or personal observances, give you mental support and balance.

The awareness and application of the yamas of nonviolence (ahimsa), truth (satya), noncovetousness (astheya), self-restraint (brahmacharya), and detachment from possessions (aparigrapha) give students of yoga the basic tools to finding balance in their interactions with the world. Most of our sense of unbalance that results in stress or depression or temporary elation stems from our interactions with the world, including the people around us. A resolve to be nonviolent, not only to others but also to our own selves, in itself fosters stability and balance. Truthfulness in speech and action, being content with our circumstances, exercising self-control, and not letting material possessions guide our thoughts and actions are practices that, when adopted in daily living, bring mental peace and balance.

The diligent practice of the niyamas of self-purification (saucha), self-contentment (santosha), self-discipline (tapas), self-study (svadhyaya), and ishvara pranidhana (self-surrender) give students a framework of concrete actions that strengthen the body and the mind, resulting in a greater sense of balance. The simple act of cleansing the body, both outwardly and inwardly, in preparation for the practice of asana fosters a sense of well-being and balance. Being content with our circumstances in life makes us aware of who we are, our goals and pursuits and what truly matters to us. Exerting the effort required in the path we choose for ourselves involves self-discipline, steadfastness and rigor. Understanding ourselves through the careful observation of our thoughts, tendencies, actions, and reactions helps us find balance in a secure sense of identity that cannot be easily shaken by how the world views us. Finally, a sense of surrender leads us to accepting ourselves and our circumstances and gives us a resolve to serve others around us. This is a powerful tool, when practiced with earnestness and sincerely, that helps bring ourselves into balance with the world.

Beyond the stage of the development of physical balance through the practice of asana, lies the stage called pranayama. This is often translated as "breath control" or "voluntary respiration." However, pranayama is more than the regulation of the breath. It is the art of utilizing the physical and physiological cue of the breath to probe, observe, and understand the mind.

Modern life has become increasingly stressful. The combined effect of technology, geopolitics, climate change, and the social culture of materialism and competitiveness makes us anxious and unbalanced. The nervous system is often depleted by overstimulation and lack of rest. The unbalanced secretion of hormones of our endocrine system, such as adrenaline and corticosterone, disrupt our digestion, sexuality, and inner reflection. Pranayama offers a practical tool to understanding the working of our minds when rigorous meditation is still out of our reach.

Although a steady practice of asana helps develop a practice of pranayama, it also fosters a subtle interplay of effort and comfort that results in a balanced, meditative state of being.

The highest stages of yoga involve pratyahara (withdrawal of the senses), dharana (concentration), dhyana (mediation), and samadhi (self-realization). These esoteric stages of yoga emerge out of a dedicated and prolonged practice of the earlier stages bringing disparate facets of the personality and the intricacies of a complex world into a state of dynamic balance.

As everyday practitioners of yoga, however, we notice that as we practice the poses, we work not only on our bodies but also on our minds. We can see the result of our efforts in our practice translate into a greater sense of comfort in our bodies. We notice an attunement to our surroundings that makes us feel more energetic and relaxed. Our emotions no longer run wild but become manageable. Our minds become capable of looking beyond the surface of things, to compartmentalize the different demands and desires of our daily lives while remaining comfortable and focused.

10. I'm an insomniac. Can yoga help me sleep better?

If your mind starts racing from one thought, plan, or emotion to another as soon as your head hits the pillow at night, you are not alone. Nearly a quarter of all working Americans are insomniacs. Not only does this mean an irretrievable opportunity for rest and rejuvenation as you lose valuable nighttime sleep, but it also results in daytime fatigue that, in turn, leads to a marked loss of productivity, increased chances for accidents and injuries, and a drastic drop in the quality of life. Specific yoga asanas and sequences help calm an overactivated nervous system, quieting the mind and priming your body to sink into a deep, restful sleep that lasts the night.

Studies show when people who suffer from insomnia perform yoga daily, their total nighttime sleep is longer, they fall asleep faster once in bed, and they return to sleep more quickly if they happen to wake up in the middle of the night. The quality and duration of out nighttime sleep usually deteriorates with age. Studies show that even for those who are sixty and older, practicing yoga regularly improves the quality and duration of sleep, making them feel better and more energized during the day. Pregnant women who have trouble sleeping due to physical discomfort also show improved quality of sleep and wake up less frequently during the night when they practice yoga in their second trimester. When cancer patients undergo chemotherapy, almost 90 percent experience insomnia. Studies show that sleep quality and duration are improved in cancer patients as well when they practice yoga regularly.

Styles of yoga such as power yoga or vigorous Vinyasa yoga are more energizing, whereas restorative yoga, yin yoga, and mindful alignment–focused yoga are more calming. The type of yoga asanas and the particular sequence of yoga asanas you practice determines the type of effect on your physical and mental state. For example, practicing a sequencing of standing poses combined with backbends energizes the body and activates the mind, making it difficult to fall asleep immediately afterward. Conversely, forward bends combined with inversions tend to quiet the body and calm the mind, promoting a sense of restfulness that is conducive to sleep.

Sirsasana (headstand), Sarvangasana (shoulder stand), Paschimottanasana (intense westward stretch), Uttanasana (intense forward stretch), Agnistambhasana (firelog pose), Uttana shishosana (extended puppy pose), Jathara parivartanasana (stomach twist pose), Viparita Karani (legs up the wall), Supta Baddha Konasana (reclining bound angle asana), and Bhastrika, Nadi Shodhan, Ujjayi II, and Chandrabhedana pranayamas together with Yoga Nidra and Shavasana are recommended for individuals who have trouble sleeping.

If you pay close attention to your breath and its effect on your mental state, you will notice that when your exhalations are long, easy, and smooth, it has a calming effect on your mind. However, when your inhalations and long, easy and smooth, it has an energizing and alerting effect on your mind. Ujjayi II pranayama, or the victorious breath, utilizes this biological phenomenon to intentionally extend the exhalation, thereby encouraging the brain and mind into a state of calm and quiet. Studies also show that Ujjayi II reduces blood pressure in individuals suffering from hypertension. As mentioned in the section on pranayama, it is strongly advisable to learn pranayama under the guidance of an experienced teacher and not by studying descriptions from a book or other media resources. This is because pranayama is a subtle, powerful practice that has the potential for causing damage as much as it can do good. It is only the watchful eye of an experienced teacher that can detect any errors in your method and practice and guide you through the journey of understanding and regulating your breath and mind.

You might also notice that during particular times of the day, it is easier to breathe through one nostril than through the other, separated by shorter phases where the breath is equally easy in both nostrils. Physiologically, a predominance of breath in the left nostril is associated with slowing down, whereas that in the right nostril is associated with speeding up of bodily functions. Chandra bhedana, or moon breath, utilizes this biological phenomenon to intentionally direct inhalations through the left nostril.

This is done using the mriga mudra. A mudra, often translated as a "seal," is a specific gesture using one or both hands and, in some cases, the whole body. A mudra aims to channel the flow of energy in the body and mind. Chandra bhedana uses the mriga mudra, or deer seal, on the right hand. This involves bending your index and middle fingers toward the palm of your hand, leaving your thumb, ring, and pinky fingers extended. In Chandra bhedana you sit in a comfortable posture, ideally in Padmasana or the lotus pose, and press the right thumb of your right hand in mriga mudra to your right nostril while inhaling deeply through your left nostril. Then you release the press of your right thumb on your right nostril and press the ring and pinky finger to your left nostril while exhaling through the right nostril. Repeating this cycle for two to three minutes brings about a distinct sense of calm and helps prepare you for a good night's sleep.

11. I have ADHD. Can yoga help me cope better?

Research shows that meditation and yoga can be very helpful in relieving symptoms of attention-deficit/hyperactivity disorder, or ADHD. A study conducted at UCLA shows ADHD patients who attended a meditation session for two and a half hours once a week and followed a home practice routine of five to fifteen minutes daily for eight weeks showed marked improvement in their ability to stay focused on tasks. Added benefits were lowering of depression and anxiety, which, in turn, further checked the symptoms of ADHD.

Studies on yoga practice in children with ADHD show increase in the levels of the feel-good biomolecule, dopamine, and increased functional connectivity in higher centers of the brain like the frontal regions of the cerebral cortex responsible for thinking, personality, decision making, and modulating social behavior. Tested on measures of attention and focus, children with ADHD who practiced yoga for at least twenty minutes twice a week over a period of eight weeks showed significant improvement.

In addition to helping with the symptoms of ADHD, yoga also benefits self-esteem, lowers stress and helps in weight loss with sustained practice. The improved brain connectivity in the higher centers of the brain indicates a greater involvement of thought before an action is taken. This in turn can reduce the amount of unhealthy food a person consumes leading to a more healthful diet.

Stress plays a major role in the acute worsening of symptoms in patients with ADHD. Increased stress in the surroundings can introduce or increase repetitive movements, inattention, impulsivity, lack of concentration, inability to follow instructions, inability to sit still and impair the patient's ability to interact with others. Studies show a decrease in stress hormones such as corticosterone and cortisol in ADHD patients who practice yoga so that they and their caregivers are better able to manage their symptoms.

Yoga asanas (physical postures), pranayama (breath work), dhyana (meditation) and chanting (mantra meditation) boost focus, confidence, and calm, helping ease the symptoms of ADHD. Chanting "Om" repeatedly has been shown to generate vibrations at a frequency of 432 Hertz where one Hertz indicates something that cycles once every second. For example, if you were to jump up and down such that you made sixty jumps in a minute, you would be jumping at a frequency of 1 Hertz. Interestingly, all things in nature and vibrations in space detected by satellites cycle at 432 Hertz. Therefore, chanting "Om" symbolically and physically tunes as into the sound of nature and the cosmos, connecting us to everything that exists. Biologically, chanting "Om" vibrates the paired vagus nerves, the most important neural highway between the brain, and several important organs such as the heart, lungs, and the digestive canal. These soothing vibrations of the vagus nerves calm the nervous system.

Most of us, including children who suffer from ADHD tend to take short, shallow breaths. Some individuals particularly affected by stress tend to hold their breath whenever confronted with a stressful situation. This can cause their faces to redden, eyes to bulge, and, in general, worsen their stress levels. Pranayama methodically increases the length of the inhalation and exhalation making the breath soft and smooth. Although generally believed to increase the blood oxygen levels, this has been contradicted by other studies that show either no sustained effect of pranayama on blood oxygen levels or an increase in carbon dioxide levels in the blood. Nevertheless, mindfully increasing the length and smoothness of the breath enhances a sense of well-being, increases energy levels, and reduces anxiety and irritability.

Balancing poses such as Tadasana (mountain pose), Vrykshasana (tree pose), Virabhadrasana III (warrior pose III), Agnisar Kriya (the roaring lion pose), forward bends, inversions, and yogic meditation techniques such as Trataka (candle gazing) and Yoganidra (yogic sleep) are calming for the nervous system and beneficial in relieving symptoms of ADHD.

12. How can yoga help me get better grades?

Acute concentration, an excellent memory, and sharp reasoning and critical thinking powers are pivotal to learning anything well and quickly.

Patanjali's Yoga Sutras, the earliest known compilation of the philosophy of yoga, defines yoga as the stilling of the fluctuations of the mind. In day-to-day parlance, that describes our ability to be attentive. Practicing yoga asanas directs our focus on our sensations at a much finer level. For example, when you're standing, you might not be attentive as to whether the weight of your body is bearing down on your toes, on the outer sides of your feet, on the inner arches of your feet or on your heels. However, when standing on one leg in tree pose, the mind is compelled to pay attention to where exactly the weight of the body is located on the sole of the standing foot. It is this sustained attention that helps bring the rest of the body into alignment so that you are, in time, able to consciously shift your center of gravity so that it can be placed right atop the heel of your standing leg. Numerous tiny movements and actions in muscles and bones, joints and fascia, throughout the body must happen consciously for you to attain the tree pose. In day-to-day life, we often put ourselves in autopilot, particularly when we are performing actions that we have performed hundreds of times before. We can sometimes read an entire passage, but because we are not paying attention, we do not understand what was actually said in the passage.

In the eightfold path of yoga, concentration is not separate from action. The subtle nature of the actions we perform in yoga asanas is a form of cultivating concentration. Yoga uses the body as a tool to access the mind. With the sustained practice of yoga asanas you develop not only the ability to sit still for extended periods, an ability that is in itself an extremely rare and difficult skill, but also the ability to withdraw your mind from external distractions like the TV blaring in the next room, and focus on the task at hand. Yoga brings the body and mind into union. In fact, the literal meaning of the word "yoga" is "addition" or "union."

Inversions such as Sirsasana (headstand) and Sarvangasana (shoulder stand) are particularly helpful in improving mental faculties. Inversions literally turn your vision upside down, giving you a different perspective on how you view the world. A change in perspective directly affects our capacity for attention. Think about when you are on vacation. The new perspective fostered by the surroundings make you see things in a new way, whereas you might not be inclined to notice things on your own street that you see every day.

Inversions, particularly Sirsasana, referred to as the king of asanas, inverts the physiology of the body, changing your blood pressure, and the pressure on your head, neck, shoulders, blood vessels, lungs, and legs. The inverted position increases blood flow to the brain, replenishing it at an increased rate with much-needed fuel and oxygen and toning the muscles that line blood vessels. Decrease in mental capacity is largely because of poor blood flow in the brain or because of the hardening of the thin vessels that carry blood to the brain, resulting in poor oxygen levels in the brain. Recent studies show that inversion therapy improves brain function by as much as 14 percent, and regular practice of inversions improves concentration, memory, powers of observation, and clarity of thought and also counteracts depression and anxiety. Moreover, some studies show that inversion therapy may play a role in arresting aging processes in the brain.

13. Which yoga poses treat adrenal fatigue and chronic stress?

Adrenal fatigue describes a group of nonspecific symptoms, including body aches, tiredness, nervousness, sleep disturbances, and digestive issues. Other symptoms include an inexplicable craving for salt and sugar and a reliance on stimulants such as caffeine. Adrenal fatigue is believed to be caused by chronic stress when the adrenal glands are no longer able to provide hormones required for the perpetually activated fight-or-flight response. It is not a bona fide medical diagnosis but, nevertheless, is a term in common circulation as well as in health books and on websites of alternative medicine. In other words, adrenal fatigue is not an accepted medical condition. The closest accepted medical term associated with suboptimal functioning of the adrenal glands is adrenal insufficiency.

Your adrenal grands are little pyramidal structures that sit atop your kidneys and secrete a variety of vital hormones, including cortisol and adrenaline. Adrenal insufficiency occurs when one or more of these vital adrenal hormones are not produced to the required level in the body. Symptoms of adrenal insufficiency include fatigue, muscle weakness, diffused aches and pains throughout the body, loss of weight and appetite for no apparent reason, low blood sugar levels, low blood pressure, dizziness or lightheadedness, hair loss, patchy discoloration of the skin, depression, and irritability. Blood tests can readily diagnose adrenal insufficiency.

What is widely agreed upon is that the adrenal glands are important in maintaining energy levels. Among the many hormones they produce is cortisol, which peaks early in the morning and then tapers off as the day progresses, reaching its lowest point at bedtime. The fall of cortisol levels synchronizes with the rise of the sleep hormone melatonin, which makes it easy to fall asleep at night. When the body senses danger, there are intense bursts of cortisol and adrenaline that trigger the fight-or-flight response. In the modern world of high stress, the body can be in constant state of alertness accompanied by lack of sleep.

For someone suffering from adrenal fatigue and its associated symptoms, it is definitely not advisable to engage in a high-energy power yoga, vinyasa flow, or hot yoga routine. A yoga sequence that is restorative and aided by props like blankets, chairs, bolsters, blocks, and straps can, on the other hand, be supportive and help you calm down. Poses where the back of the pelvis is supported and blood flow toward the adrenals is encouraged, such as Viparita Karani (legs up the wall pose) and Salamba Supta Baddha Konasana (supported reclining bound angle pose), supported Shavasana (corpse pose), and yoga nidra (yogic sleep meditation), can be extremely helpful in fostering a sense of tranquility and inner peace. The powerful technique of yoga nidra induces a state akin to deep sleep as measured by electroencephalography (EEG) but without the loss of awareness. Some students claim that a forty-five-minute practice of yoga nidra feels like sleeping for three hours. Forward-bending yoga poses, such as Adho Mukha Virasana (child's pose) and supported Paschimottanasana (intense westward stretch), also help induce a state of calm and brings relief when struck by the symptoms of adrenal fatigue.

14. Which poses prevent lower back pain?

Lower back pain can mean several different things. Lower back pain can result from muscle sprains and strains in the lumbar region of the spine when you lift something heavy from the ground while rounding your back and keeping your knees straight, so that your back bears the major brunt of the lift. Lower back pain can also result from poor posture over prolonged periods, such as sitting hunched over the computer day after day. Lower back pain can also result from certain diseases such as herniated discs, sciatica, kidney infections, infections of the spine, and abnormal spinal curvatures.

Lower back pain can negatively affect our mood and our quality of life. Careful practice of yoga asanas can prevent lower back pain and relieve aches that are already present. It is important to remember that forward bends, backward bends and twists have different effects on the spine. What type of yoga asanas will be beneficial in alleviating or preventing lower back pain depends on the particular cause of the pain. As a rule of thumb you should not practice any asana that increases your level of pain or discomfort when suffering from lower back pain. Also, sitting asanas put the maximal stress on the lower back and are best avoided when in pain.

Whereas forward bends increase the space between vertebral discs, backward bends compress the space between vertebral discs. Forward bends are generally not advisable in individuals with lower back pain, particularly the kind of lower back pain caused by hypermobile vertebral discs or slip discs. Increasing the space between the vertebral discs further in forward bends increases the risk of moving the vertebral discs out of alignment and thereby worsening the condition.

In all asanas attempted by a normal student or a person with lower back pain, it is important to maintain the normal curve of the spine. The lower spine has a natural inward dip right above the pelvis. It is important to maintain this natural curve while practicing yoga asanas and not allow the region to become flat or bulge outward.

Forward bends can be attempted if the student can maintain the natural curve of the spine with the help of props such as supporting against a wall or chair or using straps, pillows or bolsters. To avoid back pain when bending forward, ensure you are feeling the stretch in your legs while bending forward and not in your lower back. If attempting forward bends, Adho Mukha Shvanasana (downward dog pose) is a great way to lengthen the spine and decompress the spaces between the vertebral discs while maintaining the natural curvature of the spine.

Backbends should be attempted while bending from the upper back in poses such as the cobra (Bhajangasana) and the sphinx (Salamba Bhujangasana) or locust pose (Salabhasana). These asanas are found beneficial in most cases of lower back bends. However, while practicing these asanas, excessive strain should not be placed on the lower back which is generally the more flexible section of the spine and therefore easy to bend from. Care must be taken in the asana to stretch the hamstrings and the belly of the calf muscle to slowly being the heels to touch the ground. The shoulders should be moving away from the ears and toward the raised hips so that there is no compression in the neck region.

Twists are best avoided in lower back pain unless the student does not have a pinched nerve or slip disc issues. These conditions cause numbness, tingling, or sharp pain and can be easily distinguished form other causes of back pain. When assessed suitable, Jathara parivartanasana, or reclining spinal twist, is a great way to relieve tension in the entire back body in a passive way, allowing gravity to help you relax into the pose and relieve pain.

Sideways bends such as Anantasana (Vishnu's couch pose) and Utthita Parshvakonasana (extended side angle pose) are excellent ways to lengthen the spine and relieve intervertebral compressions without bending forward or backward. You should be careful to not inadvertently twist in doing sideways bends, as this can increase the pressure on the lower back.

Supine stretches such as Viparita Karani (legs-up-the-wall pose), and supine abdominal strengtheners such as Supta Padangushtasana (reclining hand to big toe pose) are also beneficial in lower back pain. When resting in Shavasana (corpse pose), it is advisable to bend the knees slightly and keep a rolled blanket or bolster under the knees if you have lower back pain.

Lower back pain can also result from sacroiliac instability. This is more common in women than in men due to the difference in the shape of the hips. The sacroiliac region is the region between the tail bone and the very top back of the thighs. Incidentally, sacroiliac instability is more common in yoga students, particularly in the West, than in the general population, suggesting that there is something in our approach to yoga asanas that makes us particularly vulnerable to this type of lower back pain. Pain at the sacroiliac joint can be avoided by paying close attention to the alignment of the pelvis in all poses, but particularly in forward bends and twists. Twists such as Marichiasana and hip-opening poses such as Baddha Konasana and Upavishta Konasana bring relief in sacroiliac pain, if done with mindful attention to keeping the pelvis (hip bone) and sacrum (tail bone) in alignment.

15. Why do I feel a "yoga high" after class?

"Yoga high" is that feeling of lingering happiness, joy, calm, and relaxation that you feel after a yoga class or a practice session in which your body, mind and spirit have been totally engrossed in the asana and the movement of the breath. It is almost a feeling of exuberance when you feel you can handle anything that life might throw at you. It is as if you've truly found your ultimate chill pill. Although it is difficult to describe the various shades of "yoga high," there is a scientific explanation to this feeling.

The flight-or-fight response is an evolutionary hand-me-down that helped our ancestors focus their mental and physical efforts to save themselves from imminent danger such as a threatening wild animal ready to pounce on them. Unfortunately, this useful flight-or-fight response cannot distinguish between life-or-death situations and everyday stress. If chronically activated over prolonged periods, this survival strategy is harmful to health as it puts unnecessary strain on the body by making the heart pound at a high rate, tensing the muscles of the limbs and the core of the body, making us sweat and effectively shutting down routine biological processes such as digestion.

The stress response begins in the brain, with the cerebral cortex detecting the stressor, the amygdala interpreting the emotion of anxiety and fear and the hypothalamus commanding the sympathetic branch of the autonomic nervous system to respond to the danger. On the other hand, the parasympathetic branch of the autonomic nervous system that generally relaxes the body's various functions is suppressed when the stress response is activated. In regulating the balance of the body, the sympathetic nervous system acts like the gas pedal while the parasympathetic system acts as the brakes in a car.

Yoga retrains the body by voluntarily generating a manageable level of stress in the body through the asanas while maintaining focus on keeping the breath long, deep, and calm. This retrains the evolutionary stress response, teaching the body that not all stress is a life-and-death situation. Effectively, subjecting the body through a progressive sequence of asanas with gradually increasing levels of difficulty, increases our threshold for stress response over time. We are able to maintain our calm even in stressful situations. The practice of asanas and pranayama also calms the sympathetic nervous system and activates the parasympathetic nervous system. Functional magnetic resonance imaging (fMRI) studies show that the interconnectivity in the brain is increased in the practice of yoga, and centers in the brain that are activated by stress, such as the amygdala, are calmed.

There are also other specific ways yoga affects the nervous system and the ability of the body to handle stress. GABA is a messenger molecule in the nervous system, a neurotransmitter, that inhibits the activity of neurons involved in fear and anxiety. Yoga increases GABA levels in the brain, as much as 27 percent in individuals who practice regularly, helping to elevate the mood and curb depression and anxiety.

In sharp contrast to what scientists believed earlier, the brain is not a static organ. Earlier, neuroscientists believed that we are born with a set of neurons that decrease and die out as we age and that there is no replacing them. But now we know, not only are new neurons constantly being born, but new wirings among neurons are formed as we develop new habits and learn new skills. This ability of the brain to change and establish new connections over time is called neuroplasticity.

Yoga influences neuroplasticity in a way that the nervous system is better able to cope with stress. In yoga you put yourself through new experiences by aligning the body in unusual ways. For example, in your attempts to get into a headstand, you carefully and voluntarily put yourself into a stressful situation. Over numerous attempts, under the watchful eye of an experienced teacher, over weeks or even years, your brain and body change to handle the stressful situation of a headstand and even progressively increase your level of calm, control, and balance while you stay in your headstand for longer periods. This organically step-by-step approach of rewiring the nervous system and retraining the body's inherent biology gives you the ability to better cope with life's stressful challenges and enhances your sense of well-being.

16. Is practicing yoga during pregnancy beneficial for delivery?

Studies report an increase in confidence and comfort and a decrease of stress and hypertension through the incorporation of yoga in prenatal care. Pregnancy is often associated with maternal depression, both during pregnancy and after delivery. This does not bode well for either the mother or the child. Yoga has become a popular nonmedicine-dependent way of addressing maternal depression during pregnancy. A large-scale study based on data pooled from six independent studies on a total of 405 pregnant women in eight different medical centers show that yoga-based interventions have a statistically significant effect in reducing pregnancy-related depression. However, most of the individual studies used in the combined analysis were preliminary studies and only considered women with mild depression.

A recent study done to assess fetal and maternal effects of practicing typical moderate-intensity yoga in the third trimester recommends yoga during this period in low-risk women. The study included twenty pregnant women between the ages of twenty-nine and thirty-five and was based on continuous monitoring of fetal and maternal heart rates and uterine activity. The study reported a significant increase in maternal heart rate during the practice of yoga, to a maximum of about 125 beats per minute, but the fetal heart rate did not change much over the course of the yoga session, although uterine activity was increased during the yoga session compared to resting time points.

Developing a prenatal yoga practice before delivery can help expectant mothers cope with anxiety associated with pregnancy, labor, and delivery. Yoga teachers profess that developing a prenatal yoga practice creates a deep connection between mother and baby and empowers a mother-to-be to listen to and trust her body. Yoga helps women remain calm and focused during the intense stress, unpredictability, and physical pain of pregnancy and delivery.

Through the practice of body-strengthening poses, hip-opening poses, and various types of breathing exercises, yoga brings about physical comfort and a capacity for concentration that stands a pregnant woman in good stead. Research shows an increase in "self-efficacy" in women who practice prenatal yoga before giving birth. Self-efficacy is defined as the level of confidence a person has in performing a task.

Studies show that the sensory perception of pain can be controlled to a large extent through the practice of yoga. Research shows that prenatal yoga helps women stay in control of their bodies and minds during the third trimester as well as during the most painful phases of pregnancy, resulting in easier and more satisfying labor and delivery experiences. An ob-gyn at a New York City hospital comments that any kind of practice in relaxation, breathing, or concentration of a point can help at the time of delivery.

Poses like the deep squat or garland pose (Malasana) strengthens the legs, lower back, and pelvic floor and also develops the skill of being able to release tension, tightness, and pain. Fear, tension and pain can have a domino effect during labor, sabotaging the body's ability to take charge of a stressful situation. Regular yoga practice allows the body to recognize stressful gripping of muscles and connective tissue in different body parts and consciously soften any gripping that occurs during labor and delivery, making the experience of delivery gentler and smoother.

Stamina and endurance are called into play when labor lasts for prolonged periods. Although studies show that in women who practice yoga regularly, the length of labor is shortened by as much as two hours, yoga also helps build stamina, helping women sustain longer labors. The

endurance and discipline one builds in holding strenuous poses for prolonged periods increases stamina, strength, and mental focus.

Breathing becomes particularly challenging in late pregnancy and
during delivery. A regular practice of pranayama increases lung capacity and develops conscious control on the largely involuntary process of
breathing, which in turn provides a tool to regulate one's reactions.

Yoga poses also foster the opening of the pelvic bones and ligaments and
help optimally position the baby for birth. Most birthing centers require
the baby's head to point downward for a natural vaginal birth. Some yoga
poses, such as pelvic tilts, practiced under the guidance of an experienced
teacher and correctly timed, encourage a baby in breech or posterior position to turn in the uterus such that its head directs downward.

Physicians, therapists, and yoga teachers caution that yoga should not
be used as a means to pressure women or convince oneself into winning
some contest for pain endurance during pregnancy. Pregnancy and labor
are highly stressful experiences with every woman's personal experience
being different from any textbook case study. Yoga's reassuring benefit lies
in helping us be present in the moment and cope with the gamut of experiences and emotions that life throws at us.

17. Will yoga help me get better at sports?

Different sports usually place specific demands on particular muscle
groups and distinct parts of our anatomy, as well as overall demands on our
strength, flexibility, balance, endurance, and mental capacities. For example, running a marathon places specific demands on our leg and spine
muscles while also challenging our lung capacity, stamina, and focus.
Baseball places specific demands on shoulder muscles and joints and also
requires excellent hand-eye coordination and fast reflexes. Above all,
all sports pose the risk for injuries, and yoga helps in putting you back
together on your path to recovery. Coaches of different kinds of sports say
from personal experience that yoga enhances any athletic performance,
helps prevent injury, and in the event of injury, helps in the recovery
process.

Certain yoga asanas that are particularly helpful for athletes include
Urdhva Dhanurasana, or wheel pose, which increases arm strength,
opens the back body, shoulders, and hips; Adho Mukha Shvanasana,
or downward-facing dog pose, which stretches the backs of the legs and
increases arm strength; Gadudasana, or eagle pose, which fosters balance and stability while opening the hips and shoulders; and Baddha

Virabhadrasana, or humble warrior pose, which opens the hips and shoulders while strengthening the legs.

Flexibility is a requirement in many different sports, whether baseball, running, cycling, or cheerleading. Yoga gradually increases your range of motion by working at the levels of the bones, muscles, and fascia or connective tissue. This greatly benefits sports that require swinging actions such as tennis, golf, and so on. Increased flexibility also helps prevent injury.

We usually think of building strength in terms of lifting weights. However, yoga uses your progressive ability to lift your own body weight to build strength. This avoids injuries that occur out of the rush to lift weights you are not ready for.

Balance in yoga is not simply a physical action or movement, it is a mental approach and can even be described as a lifestyle. Yoga allows the gradual development of balance by teaching us to be gentle with ourselves and go with the flow. Yoga teaches us to take ourselves—our bodies, our experiences, our thoughts and opinions—lightly, with a sense of humor. The lightness of yoga poses that develops through persistent practice slowly permeates into other arenas of life. It is this holistic approach to life that allows a yogi to hold a headstand or stand on one leg for extended periods.

The ease of movement that yoga brings about in particularly helpful in endurance sports like long-distance running, triathlons, and Iron Mans. Yoga helps you tune into your body and mind and teaches you how to pace yourself for the long haul. It transforms your approach to sports from the level of a competition to a meditation.

Core strength is needed in almost all kinds of sports. Some yoga poses that help develop core strength include Salabhasana (locust pose), Vashishthasana (side plank pose), Navasana (boat pose), Virabhadrasana III (warrior III pose), Urdhva Prasarita Padasana (upward extension of legs pose), and Ardha Pincha Mayurasana (dolphin pose).

Postural stability in a key concern in preventing falls and fractures. A recent study on a population at high risk for postural instability showed that the regular practice of gentle yoga over eight weeks improved postural stability. The sessions included yoga stretches and simple movements in coordination with breathing, poses involving movements of major muscle groups, joint rotations, self-massage, twisting poses, standing poses, sun salutation, deep relaxation in Shavasana (corpse pose), and breathing exercises. The effect of individual yoga sessions can however be transient. It is in developing a regular daily personal practice that students develop postural grace and stability.

Recovery from sports-related injuries can be a long-drawn-out and painful affair. Yoga can help in the recovery process. In instances of plantar fasciitis commonly seen in sports that involve running and jumping, such as soccer, football, golf, tennis, and volleyball, sitting in modified Vajrasana (thunderbolt pose) with the toes tucked under and the sides of the big toes touching each other, targets the muscles and connective tissue in the sole of the foot while stretching the calf muscles that moves the toes and supports the arch of the foot. Supta padangushtasana (reclining hand-to-big-toe pose) also helps loosen and relieve the sole of the foot by stretching the hamstrings and the tissues that run along the back of the hip, thigh, and calf. When the sole of the foot gets tight, these muscles and connective tissue tug on the sole of the foot, increasing the discomfort.

Yoga changes the way you think about yourself and the world around you. Yoga increases your sensitivity to perceive subtle sensations in your own body as well as stimuli from your environment. Increase in ease of movement and decrease in forceful effort not only shifts your perspective over time but also prevents injuries.

18. What impact does yoga have on flexibility? Do I need to be flexible to do yoga?

Physicians and physical therapists recognize flexibility to be the third pillar of fitness, next to cardiovascular health and strength. Flexibility is central to achieving optimal health and may play a role in preventing injury and more serious illnesses such as arthritis and depression.

Flexibility depends on the efficient working of muscles, tendons, ligaments, joints, and bones. Flexibility is also a medically used diagnostic indicator for health. Studies have shown that age and stressful situations such as homelessness decrease a person's flexibility. Yoga therapists generally assess flexibility by measuring the distance a person can reach while sitting (sit and reach test), the ability to bring the soles of the feet together while sitting as in Baddha Konasana, and the ability to twist the trunk.

When muscles lengthen, the connective fibers that connect those muscles to the bones, called tendons, also stretch. The increase in muscle strength is proportional to the length to which the tendons can stretch. Therefore, flexible tendons increase your capacity for muscle strength. Flexibility combined with aerobic fitness allows you to adapt to different physical stressors. Otherwise, common bad habits such as hunching over your phone or computer screen or the natural loss of muscular elasticity with age can make you feel so stiff that any sudden awkward motion could potentially lead to injury. Flexibility improves blood circulation through your muscles and keeps the walls of your arteries pliable, helping keep a host of diseases at bay, such as diabetes, kidney disease, stroke and heart attack.

One of the main reasons people hesitate to practice yoga is the fear of not being flexible enough. However, yoga doesn't need you to be flexible although yoga is often culturally distorted as involving moves that twist you into a pretzel. The purpose of yoga is to find inner peace and stillness through mindful practice of asanas and breathing. In the process of achieving this you increase your bodies flexibility in balance with your strength and lung capacity.

Though there are many different styles and schools of yoga, each path works from the inside out and makes you work at your capacity while still pushing your edge. Traditions like the Iyengar school use props such as wooden blocks, straps and bolsters to help those of us who are not flexible enough for a particular asana, to still benefit maximally from it. Other schools such as Bikram yoga use heat to help you stretch your muscles.

Yoga is not about competing but about going within to understand the range of motion of your own body and mind. Each time you practice yoga you create muscle memory and pathways in your neural network that act as a launchpad for your next practice.

In fact, many yoga teachers are of the opinion that it is safer to be inflexible than hyperflexible as a beginner student in yoga. Individuals with hyperflexible joints are more prone to injure themselves in attempting a new asana than inflexible individuals.

Flexibility is also important for athletics and strenuous sports such as cycling. It is no surprise that spin classes include a stretching regimen. Stretching in simple and gentle yoga asanas before and after athletic sports increases the range of motion in your joints and prevents injury. Stretching also warms up muscles and increases blood flow in the hip flexors, hamstrings, and quadriceps before strenuous running sessions.

19. Is yoga a good way to improve muscle strength?

There is a lot of controversy as to whether yoga can replace strength training or whether it should be complemented by strength training. Conventionally strength training is carried out using weights as resistance with multiple repetitions of each muscle group. Medical practitioners recommend strength training at least twice a week, not only to keep the metabolic machinery in tune but also to prevent bone loss. Bone loss coupled with vitamin D deficiency fostered through our increasingly indoor and sedentary lifestyle is common in the U.S. population, even among children.

Yoga does not use weight machines, dumbbells, or resistance cords. Instead it uses the weight of your own body as the resistance against which you gradually build up your strength. This has the advantage of reducing or even eliminating chances of injury through the lifting of weights that are beyond your capacity. In yoga, as you work your body into different asanas, you must support these new and unusual orientations using the strength of different groups of muscles.

In traditional schools of yoga, a student generally begins with standing poses. This allows the strengthening of the legs—the foundation of all standing poses—before the student progresses to forward bends, backbends, twists, arms balances and inversions. Building from the foundation upward in all asanas is one of the core features in the traditional teachings of yoga. Standing poses such as Trikonasana (triangle pose); Utthita Parshva Konasana (extended side angle pose); Virabhadrasana I, II, and III (warrior poses 1, 2, and 3); and Utkatasana (fierce pose) are great ways to strengthen your legs, torso, and even your arms before incorporating more difficult strength-building poses into your practice.

In addition to a strong foundation, it is also important to build core strength. Yoga does this in a gradual and graded manner so that you strengthen your core without undue risks of internal disbalance, strain, or injury. Asanas such as Navasana (boat pose), Chaturanga dandasana (four-limbed staff pose), and Ardha Pincha Mayurasana (dolphin pose) are great ways to strengthen your core in yoga.

Another advantage in attempting to develop strength through the practice of yoga is that even if the body is not strong enough for a particular asana, benefits can still be gained through the practice of intermediate postures and through the judicious use of props under the guidance of an able teacher. For example, when a student is not strong enough to kick up both legs onto the wall in a full arm balance or hand stand (Adho Mukha Vrkshasana, literally, downward-facing tree pose), the student can still be guided to lift both legs onto a chair or even walk both legs up the wall and practice an L-shaped pose until the arms and shoulders have gained enough strength to kick up into a handstand.

Arm balances such as Bakasana (crane pose), Bhujapidasana (shoulder-pressing pose), and Ashtavakrasana (eight-angled pose) are justifiably meant for the advanced student who has developed the strength in the arms and spine to lift his or her own weight in these poses. Before one attempts these asanas that demand a high degree of strength, the student usually practices simpler arm balances such as Adho Mukha Shvanasana (downward-facing dog pose), wherein a large portion of the body's weight is placed on the arms.

Counterintuitively, inversions are taught fairly early on in the progressive teachings of yoga, though still after some mastery of the standing poses has been achieved. Inversions definitely require upper body and arm strength; however, they also involve the development of a sense of balance, which counteracts the strength and effort exerted in the inversions with a sense of ease and effortlessness.

20. Is yoga beneficial for losing weight?

If you're looking for a way to lose weight fast, yoga is not the way to go. Developing a daily yoga practice does, over time, alter your metabolism, balancing your metabolic rate to the level and intensity of your yoga practice and lifestyle. However, the gradual, progressive method of traditional yoga teaching is not suitable for or aimed at rapid weight loss.

Scientific studies show that a ninety-minute session of Bikram yoga or hot yoga, one of the more intense form of yoga practices, burns an average of 286 kcal. Inexperienced students have been shown to burn fewer calories than experienced students in identical yoga sessions. Ninety-minute Bikram yoga sessions led inexperienced yoga students to burn on average 3.7 kcal per kilogram of body weight, whereas experienced students burnt on average 4.7 kcal per kilogram of body weight. The American College of Sports Medicine classifies this as light-to-moderate-intensity exercise. Theoretically, light-to-moderate-intensity physical practices can be used for weight maintenance or weight loss if practiced several times a week.

Sun salutations, a cyclical series of postures that are an integral aspect of Hatha yoga is commonly practiced in many traditional and modern schools of yoga. A scientific study shows that a thirty-minute session of sun salutations burns on average 230 kcal in individuals with a mean body weight of 60 kilograms or 132 pounds.

Active, intense styles of yoga practices such as Bikram, Vinyasa, and power yoga burn more calories than less intense forms of yoga such as Restorative or Yin yoga. However, over extended practice, all forms of yoga affect the body's metabolism. An NIH-funded study shows Restorative yoga burns subcutaneous fat, or the layer of fight right under the skin, in overweight women with a body mass index (BMI) of 30 or more. The study compared clinically obese women who participated in either a forty-eight-week restorative yoga session or one performing stretching exercises. Both groups showed weight loss, but the restorative yoga group lost 2.5 times the amount of subcutaneous fat as the group performing stretching exercises. The study also showed that whereas the stretching exercise group regained much of the lost weight after six months, the restorative yoga group continued to lose weight after six months.

In addition to gradual but long-lasting metabolic change and weight loss, yoga brings about an overall behavioral change, including a change in eating habits, sleeping patterns, and enhancing mindfulness and focus in daily activities. The combined effect of all these changes affects the body weight over extended periods of practice.

If you intend to use your yoga practice for weight loss, you could begin your journey by focusing on these asanas that not only help you burn fat, particularly when held for extended periods, but also help you build muscle tone and enhance your flexibility: Navasana (boat pose), Utthita Parshva Konasana (extended side-angle pose), Chaturanga Dandasana (four-limbed staff pose), Marichiasana I (pose dedicated to Sage Marichi, I), Paschimottanasana (seated forward bed pose or intense extension-of-the-west pose), Purvottanasana (intense extension-of-the-east pose), Urdhva Mukha Shvanasana (upward-facing dog pose), Utkatasana (fierce pose or chair pose) and Virabhadrasana II (warrior pose II).

Risks and Concerns

21. What should I do if I feel physical discomfort or pain in a yoga pose?

Yoga not only stretches the muscles you use frequently in your day-to-day activities but also reaches deep into your muscular, skeletal, and connective tissue to contract and relax them deeply and in unusual and unfamiliar ways. Therefore, it is no surprise if you develop some discomfort including mild to moderate levels of body ache and soreness either immediately after your yoga practice or even twelve to forty-eight hours after your practice. Moreover, sometimes muscles can also feel sore upon overuse.

Though yoga is generally thought of as a low-impact exercise, when practiced with focus and devotion, it is capable of reaching deep into your physical and mental core, challenging your capacity, strength, endurance, and flexibility in different ways. Therefore, all yoga practitioners, whether novices or experienced students, experience some discomfort and soreness from time to time. When the body moves in unusual ways, it causes microinjuries to the muscle and connective tissues, which trigger the body's inflammatory response. This causes muscle soreness. Over time the muscle soreness heals resulting in enhanced muscle development and functional capacity. However, if you develop extreme, unbearable pain after your yoga class or practice, you should see a doctor immediately.

If the soreness is minimal and bearable, you could take several steps to ease your discomfort while your body recovers. Staying hydrated helps increase the total volume of blood that circulates through your body, allowing blood to flow easily through the muscles to transfer nutrition, remove pain-causing metabolic wastes like lactic acid, and heal the cells. It is best to hydrate by drinking water and not caffeine or energy drinks. Caffeine and energy supplements add unnecessary calories and can increase pain perception.

Getting adequate sleep is also central to the body's healing process. During sleep, the body's nervous system goes into the rest-and-digest mode, and the hormones target the body's tissues that need repair and relaxation.

Taking a hot bath also helps activate the body's rest-and-digest nervous system. This minimizes the stress and tension on the body and allows the natural healing process to begin.

It is important to continue gentle exercises during the period that you are feeling sore. Gentle exercise after yoga relieves soreness, relaxes muscle spasms and allows muscles, connective tissue and joints to heal and develop their functional capacity. For example, using a foam roller for about twenty minutes after a yoga practice session reduces tenderness in the long run, even if it causes some immediate discomfort. It's important to remember to stretch in all planes of motion during the healing period to increase blood circulation, prevent stress and pain, and increase your range of motion. Intense stretching during the healing period, however, is not beneficial and can do more harm than good.

A balanced meal after your yoga practice helps repair microinjuries in the muscular and skeletal systems. Nourishment also speeds up the recovery process, shortening the duration of your soreness after a yoga session.

It is not advisable to take anti-inflammatory medications to curb your soreness after yoga. The body's natural inflammatory pathways help repair damaged tissue. If you prevent the body's normal inflammation by taking anti-inflammatory drugs, you are curbing your body's ability to heal itself.

Finally, though counterintuitive, one of the best ways to tackle yoga-induced soreness is to do more yoga, but gently. If you concentrate on the painful or sore areas, directing your breath and mental focus to these area to slowly relieve the tightness and tension, it is more beneficial in the long run than not moving at all because you're sore. If your range of motion in a certain area is limited due to soreness, continue to gently direct your attention and breath to that area while you practice the same yoga poses that you did before but in a more relaxed and gentle manner.

This will not only help you overcome your soreness quicker but help you increase the strength and function of that region of your body.

22. Why do my joints pop during practice?

If your fingers or knees make a clicking, cracking, or popping noise in some yoga poses or even in your day-to-day activities, you are not alone. You might have heard people warning you that if you crack your knuckles, they might get bigger—or worse, you might develop arthritis. Although these common notions are largely myths, some forms of cracking or popping joints are not desirable. The seriousness of any sound associated with movements while practicing yoga—whether it's a pop, crackle, snap, or crunch—depends on the cause of the sound.

No one knows exactly why joints crack and pop. One theory holds that gases, most commonly nitrogen, which are trapped in the synovial fluid that surrounds a joint, escape from the fluid in the joint when the joint is pushed into or out of its normal position. This can cause a popping sound. Another reason for the noise is believed to be the movement of connective tissue that hold joints and muscles together, ligaments and tendons, over the joints. Yet another reason for audible movements can be arthritis that sets in the joints from the erosion of cartilage that pads the surface of contact between bony areas in a joint, causing bones to rub together. When bones rub together, it causes friction, which results in a popping sound, much like when you snap your thumb and index finger hard enough to generate friction.

Clinicians, osteopaths, and yoga experts believe that if sounds occur naturally in day to day activities or while practicing yoga and there is no pain associated with the noise, it is not a concern. However, to forcibly pop one's own joints, like cracking your knuckles frequently, is not advisable. Intentionally cracking your joints can lead to hypermobility and instability of the joint and can cause the muscles in the vicinity to strain to support the joint, leading cyclically to an increase the urge to crack the joints again.

On the other hand, if the sound in the joint arises from a tendon or ligament moving over the joint, it is best to monitor it closely, and if pain or swelling increases at any point, it is recommended to seek help from a qualified health professional at the earliest.

The knee joint is particularly prone to making audible creaking noises in poses such as Utkatasana (or the chair pose or fierce pose) when you squat with your feet and knees together and a high degree of pressure is placed on the joint. Another pose where you frequently encounter a popping sound is when you're coming out of Chatushpadasana (or bridge pose). In the case of Utkatasana the feet can be placed hip width apart instead of together, as in the classical pose, to reduce the pressure on the knee joint and any resulting creaking sounds. In Chatushpadasana, when you are coming out of the pose and lying on your back, the knees make and acute angle between the backs of the shin, or calves, and the thighs and this puts a high degree of flexion stress on the knee joint. Increasing the angle between the calves and the back of the thighs can reduce the flexion of the knee in Chatushpadasana and reduce or prevent any noise. In order to increase the angle between the back thighs and calves, move the feet away from the hips while coming out of the pose.

In the practice of yoga, when your skeletal framework is adopting unusual positions, causing your joints to make curious noises. If these noises are minimal and not accompanied by any pain whatsoever, you have nothing to worry about. However, if these noises are caused due to overloading the joints or due to poor alignment, these noises might be a warning signal to take a step back and pay closer attention to the cause.

23. Why do I get dizzy during yoga?

Low blood sugar levels and dehydration are the primary causes of dizziness during a yoga session. Withholding natural bodily functions such as the urge to urinate or pass gas can also result in spells of dizziness.

According to Ayurveda, an Indian form of medicine and a sister discipline of yoga, dizziness is linked to vata dosha. Dosha is a Sanskrit word that is most commonly translated as biological energies or biological constitution. According to the principals of Ayurveda, everybody has a unique combination of the three primary doshas: kapha, pitta, and vata. A body type that is predominated by kapha has more of the water and earth elements. A body type that is predominantly pitta has more of the fire and water elements. And a body type that is primarily vata has more of the space and air element. As per Ayurvedic principles, when the three forms of bioenergy are in balance with each other, one feels energetic, creative, adaptable, enterprising, and expressive. However, when vata is out of balance, one feels scattered, anxious, overwhelmed, restless; digests food poorly; and is frequently constipated and suffers from insomnia. Skipping meals, working or staying awake long hours into the night, and withholding natural urges aggravate the vata dosha.

If you are assessed to be prone to aggravated vata dosha, you might find yourself frequently dizzy during or after yoga sessions. One way of managing these spells of dizziness is to always honor nature's calls to defecate, urinate, pass gas, sneeze, yawn, or cough. To forcibly withhold these urges due to pressures at work or social etiquettes can cause the vata bioenergy to become imbalanced, manifesting in forms such as dizziness.

Maintaining regular routines for daily activities, particularly eating, working, and sleeping, is calming to the vata bioenergy. When attending yoga classes, this means, you need to time your yoga classes around your eating routine. It is not advisable to eat anything in the couple of hours leading up to your yoga class. Yoga asanas and pranayama are best practiced on an empty stomach and after you have cleared your bowels. However, it is important to find your own balance of nutrition and hydration so that you have enough strength for your practice but are not feeling stuffed, bloated, or uncomfortable. Eating a light, balanced meal a couple of hours before yoga class gives you a sufficient time window to digest your food before your class.

Restorative yoga poses are best suited for individuals prone to dizziness. Grounding asanas such as Supta Baddha Konasana (reclined bound angle pose) and Supta Virasana (reclined victor's pose) are good to incorporate into your practice if you feel dizzy during a yoga class. Switching to a slower yoga style that focuses more on alignment and holding poses for longer times rather than switching from one pose to another in quick succession, is recommended for those who experience dizziness while practicing yoga. Avoiding hot yoga, standing forward bends, and unsupported inversions is also recommended for those prone to dizziness. Being mindful of your alignment in all yoga poses you practice, having your eyes open while practicing yoga to utilize visual cues optimally, and developing a pranayama practice help in refining the sensibilities to a level that any dizziness can be detected at the very beginning, preventing any injuries during your yoga practice caused by falling due to dizziness.

Practicing pranayama also can lead to spells of dizziness, particularly when blood oxygen and carbon dioxide levels vary radically from your normal physiological capacity due to the breath you are practicing. The brain is the highest consumer of oxygen in the body. When blood oxygen levels fall and carbon dioxide levels rise, it can lead to dizziness. Being extremely careful, particularly when you are first learning pranayama is critical in avoiding dizziness and other side effects of a hasty technique. Learning from an experienced teacher and being highly vigilant to how your body reacts to each type of pranayama will avoid any experience of unwanted side effects during pranayama, such as dizziness.

24. Why do my muscles shake or tremble during yoga?

Whether you are a beginner at yoga or an experienced practitioner, when you are in a yoga asana, you can sometimes experience involuntary vibration, shaking, or trembling in your muscles at various degrees of intensity.

Oftentimes this trembling is associated with a pose that you would consider physically demanding that requires a great deal of physical strength and effort on your part. Arm balances such as Adho Mukha Vrykshasana (handstand pose or downward-facing tree pose) or Bakasana (crane or crow pose) would fall into this category.

However, asanas that do not require intense effort, but for which the body is in an unusual orientation can also cause vibrations, shaking or trembling. Inversions such as Sirsasana (Head stand pose) and Sarvangasana (shoulder stand pose) would fall under this category. Although initially effortful, once headstand and shoulder-stand poses are mastered they are calming and quieting to the senses and are maintained by the practitioner more from a sense of balance than from active muscular effort. Despite the calming intention of these inversions, they can sometimes lead to subtle, moderate or intense shaking.

Paradoxically, restful restorative poses can also lead to shaking and trembling if held for prolonged periods. Poses such as Baddha Konasana (bound angle pose or cobbler's pose) or Supta Virasana (supine victor's pose) would be examples of restorative poses that if held for a long time can lead to trembling.

In physically strenuous asanas, quivering muscles are a physiological and neurological signal of muscular fatigue and exhaustion. In certain conditions, where there is minimal chance of injury, yoga teachers may suggest holding such poses through the shaking while being mindful of your alignment and maintaining your focus on your breath. However, if your focus on the alignment of the asana falters, or you are in a balance pose falling out of which can be injurious, yoga teachers suggest coming out of the pose safely as soon as you experience any shaking or trembling.

The breath is a wonderful yardstick that can be used by yoga students as a measure of their capacity for holding a particular asana. Ancient yoga texts mention that, ideally, a yoga asana should balance effort and ease. While in a difficult yoga pose, you should still be able to inhale and exhale smoothly. If you find you cannot inhale and exhale smoothly, your breath is becoming shallow to the point that you are feeling suffocated, or if you are holding your breath, your body has likely reached the limit of its capacity, and it is time you come out of the pose.

Dehydration is another common cause of muscular quivering. Lack of adequate water can disbalance electrolytes like sodium and potassium that carry electrical impulses along nerves and allow your muscles to contract. It is a good idea to drink water two to three hours before a yoga practice session that lasts for an hour or more. This will ensure that your body has enough water to maintain your electrolyte balance despite the moisture you might lose through sweating during your yoga practice.

Yoga fosters balance and equilibrium in the body by exerting effort in the musculoskeletal system and at the same time calming the body through a focus on deep and smooth breathing. In beginners and even advanced students, this contradictory approach can sometimes lead to a clash between the primitive part of the brain that has evolved to sense danger and trigger the flight-or-fight response or survival mode and the part of the brain that seeks to maintain status quo. When you are in a difficult yoga pose, the intense muscular effort and danger of possible injury can signal your body to be in survival model while the mindful breathing can induce a sense of safety and relaxation. These two opposing forces can sometimes trigger an energy release that is manifested in the form of vibrations that either localize to a specific part of the anatomy or run through the entire body.

25. Why am I not supposed to eat two to three hours before yoga practice? How do I manage my diet to get maximum benefit from my yoga practice?

Why one should not eat two to three hours before yoga practice or any strenuous exercise or sleep for that matter has a very simple and logical explanation and is not simple a blind ritual. The body functions optimally when it is able to utilize the available energy throughout the day. Regular mealtimes therefore train the body to anticipate energy intake and maintains steady biological rhythms. Digestion of food itself requires a high expenditure of energy. Avoiding food two to three hours before yoga ensures that the energy required for digestion is not taken away for the physical and mental effort needed in the practice of yoga. Now if you have an extremely fast metabolism, you might be able to digest your meal in shorter times and can therefore decrease the time window between your meal and your yoga practice. On the other hand, if you have an extremely slow metabolism, you might need more time to digest your food and should increase the time between your meal and yoga practice. On average, a two- to three-hour period between a moderate meal and the start of your yoga practice is sufficient to digest your food.

There are a lot of diet fads out there that tell us what to eat and when, from farm-raised fish, grass-fed beef diets to organic, vegan, gluten-free, and macrobiotic diets. A yogic diet, however, follows some broad and simple rules that can be incorporated into whatever your specific choice of diet might be. According to yogic and Ayurvedic principles, food choices are based on the individual's constitution, on the current requirements of his life, and on the season. Nourishing the body properly is central to physical and mental health and progress along the path of yoga.

Yoga and Ayurveda classify food as tamasic, rajasic, or sattvic. Tamasic foods are those with a pungent odor that leave us feeling dull and heavy and that are difficult to digest. Onions, meat, and garlic are considered tamasic food. Rajasic foods can either promote dullness or hyperactivity and include foods such as coffee, hot peppers, and salt. Sattvic foods tend to keep the body feeling light and the mind clear. These include fresh fruits and vegetables, whole grains, seeds, legumes, milk, and milk products. The food choices that are best for you would be based on your constitution, known in Sanskrit as vikriti, and your current state or nature, known in Sanskrit as prakriti. Moreover, a yogic diet also takes into consideration the yama or universal principle of ahimsa or nonviolence. As such, most yogis and yoginis follow a vegetarian or vegan diet.

According to yoga philosophy, every living being is a multilayered entity. Layers in Sanskrit are koshas. The grossest layer of our beings is Annamaya Kosha, literally the layer of food. This constitutes our physical bodies. Therefore, for yogis food choices reflect personal ethics, current physical requirements, and harmony with their surroundings. The food we ingest is what our physical body is made of and is central to the state and manifestation of our life force, or prana shakti.

26. Is it safe to practice inversions?

Inversions are yoga poses that orient your body upside down. Technically, all asanas where the heart and the hips are above the head are labeled inversions. By this definition, some of the simplest inversions are Balasana, or child's pose; Uttanasana, or forward fold; Viparita Karani, or legs up the wall pose; and Adho Mukha Shvanasana, or downward-facing dog pose. More challenging inversions in yoga include Adho Mukha Vrykshasana (downward-facing tree pose or handstand), Ardha

Pincha Mayurasana (dolphin pose), Pincha Mayurasana (forearm balance or feathered peacock pose), Halasana (plow pose), Sarvangasana (shoulder stand); and, of course, Sirsasana (headstand).

Going upside down brings up a lot of fear issues. Working with this fear, understanding your fear, and observing your fears are part of your yoga practice or self-study (Svadhyaya). From the time of learning to crawl and walk in childhood, we've mostly lived our waking lives with our feet on the ground and our heads held high. Reversing this orientation therefore is understandably unusual, uncomfortable, and scary. It forces you out of your comfort zone and literally turns your world upside down.

Even a beginner yoga student is introduced to inversions in Uttanasana and Adho Mukha Shvanasana. These inversions, though apparently simple, train the body and mind to reorient upside down. Adho Mukha Shvanasana begins to train the arm muscles and skeletal alignment that is needed to attempt more difficult inversions.

Safety in inversions is largely dependent on the individual's physical and mental state. That is why it is so important to learn inversions from an experienced teacher. A qualified teacher is able to gauge your level of strength and the precision of your alignment and guide you through gradual progressions into inversions, minimizing the risks of falling or injury. Even advanced yoga students who practice inversions every day find that their stability, steadiness, and comfort in inversions vary from day to day. Our bodies change subtly from day to day due to a variety of factors and therefore respond differently to inversions. If there is any shaking or unsteadiness, even advanced students are advised to come out of their inversions or not attempt inversions for the day.

Individuals with spine issues such as scoliosis, neck or head injuries, or high blood pressure or cardiovascular issues must take extra caution in inversions. Generally, persons who take medications to keep high blood pressure under control can still practice the same inversions as a person with normal blood pressure, taking care to progress gradually under the guidance of an able teacher.

Warming up your arm muscles, hips, and spine, paying close attention to your musculoskeletal alignment, progressing in a step-by-step manner, and refining your ability and focus to listen to the subtle cues from your body all increase safety in practicing inversions. Beginners are usually guided into inversions through simpler poses and with the use of props such as a chair or the wall. For example, Viparita Karani (legs up the wall pose), in which your hips are lifted up on a stack of blankets or a bolster, your shoulders and head are on the ground, and your legs and sitting bones are flush against the wall, is a good way to stabilize and strengthen the body as well as get the feel of being inverted, without the need for arm strength or any risk of falling.

You should only attempt standing on your head after you have been practicing yoga under the guidance and supervision of a suitable teacher for at least a few years. Use the wall. Your first attempts at headstand should be at the wall. This teaches you when you are truly aligned and prevents falls.

The most common risk of standing on your head is injury to the cervical spine and damage to the eyes. You can reduce the risk of hurting your neck in headstand by first developing shoulder strength and alignment. Practicing holding these four poses for at least two minutes each helps train your shoulders and develops your proprioception for correct alignment: downward dog, wide-legged forward bend, forearm plank, dolphin pose.

To relieve tension on your neck muscles and cervical spine, practice these three poses consecutively following every headstand or attempt at headstand: child's pose, downward dog, and standing forward and bending while holding your elbows (also known as dangling pose).

If headstand is considered the father of all asanas, shoulder stand is veritably the mother of all asanas. Learn shoulder stand before you attempt headstand. You can practice shoulder stand without practicing headstand, but whenever you practice headstand, it is advisable to follow it up with a practice of shoulder stand. Headstand has a heating effect on the body and mind that is reversed by shoulder stand.

Inversions are refreshing, energizing, and invigorating. They counteract the effects of gravity on an upright posture and are considered a panacea for common musculoskeletal, nervous, and hormonal ailments. Inversions are extremely beneficial not only in boosting our confidence and self-esteem, increasing our attention, and reducing bouts anxiety and depression but also in giving our hearts a rest from constantly pumping freshly oxygenated blood to meet the demands of the brain. Inversions have been proven to reduce blood pressure and heart rate and improve the working of the circulatory and lymphatic systems. Inversions are also highly energizing and build a stronger and more balanced core.

27. Should I practice yoga if I'm on my period?

During the monthly period, it is best to either take a rest from yoga practice or undertake an easy, relaxed, and restorative practice avoiding undue effort and strain. However, the practice of certain yoga asanas and pranayamas can bring relief from discomfort and disorders related to the menstrual cycle, and they can still be practiced during one's period.

Adolescence is a period of great changes, when the body and mind transitions from childhood to maturity. The start of the menstrual cycle during adolescence is accompanied by changes in the pituitary gland—a small, pea-sized organ that acts as the master regulator of major body functions, including menstruation. Starting yoga practice before or during the onset of menstruation helps the body and mind through this period of growth and transition with equanimity, strength, and mental poise. Inversions stimulate the pituitary gland. In addition, forward bends are helpful in massaging the abdominal organs, improving circulation and resulting oxygenation in the region of the ovaries and uterus. Practicing standing poses during periods promotes strength, balance, and skeletal growth.

Some women suffer from various menstruation-related disorders that include both physical and mental symptoms. Due to conditions such as hormonal imbalances, malnutrition, or anxiety, the menstrual cycle can be delayed or absent (amenorrhea), light or infrequent (oligomenorrhea), or accompanied by severe physical and mental discomfort prior to menstruation (premenstrual syndrome). Practicing yoga releases endorphins, which elevate the mood and help counter mood swings, anxiety, and depression, which can occur before or during the menstrual cycle at varying degrees of severity. Practicing yoga during your period also helps calm the nervous system, easing stress and encouraging deep relaxation in the body and mind.

According to yogic traditions, the time of menstruation is predominated by an emphasis of apana vayu in the body, which essentially indicates a downward flow of energy. Yogis down the ages, through carefully observing the body and breath, came to the conclusion that the essential life force of the body (prana) can be divided into five components. These they named vayus or winds. By bringing awareness to the vayus, yogis seek to cultivate conscious control of the flow of the five vayus that leads to optimal health and well-being. Each vayu is primarily connected to a specific region of the body and is associated with specific bodily functions. However, they are interdependent and function in synchrony. Prana vayu is located in the chest and is associated with intake of food, breath, and forward movement. Apana vayu, located in the pelvis, is associated with elimination of waste from the body, and downward and outward movement. Samana vayu, located in the navel region, is associated with assimilation, discernment, inner absorption, and consolidation. Udana vayu, located in the throat region, is associated with speech, expression, and upward movement. Vyana vayu is dispersed through the whole body and is associated with circulation, expansiveness, and spreading.

During menstruation, when the body is removing the unfertilized lining of the uterus, the predominant flow of energy is downward and outward. This is why many yoga teachers advise against inversions, that is, any pose where the heart is above the level of the head, including downward-facing dog pose, bridge pose, plow pose, wheel pose, shoulder stand, handstand, and headstand. Inversions promote the body's energy to move upward, leading to a predominance of prana vayu in the chest and udana vayu in the throat. So, practicing inversions can create stress and other disorders in the body by inducing an imbalance through the predominance of an upward mobile energy when the body's natural energy flow is downward.

According to yogic and ayurvedic texts, menstruation is a time for cleansing and rejuvenating. Spending time in silence, rest and reflection helps the mind and body through this phase. Yoga teachers therefore advise to listen to your body very carefully and based on your observations, either practice gentle yoga, or practice certain poses that alleviate pain or adopt a more energetic practice if the body feels stiff and dull.

Mainstream medical science, however, does not yet acknowledge the subtle flow of energy in the body to the extent discussed in yogic and ayurvedic texts. The basis of medical concerns regarding inversions stem from the possibility that they may cause retrograde menstruation, a condition where the blood moves upward rather than downward, and lead to endometriosis. Endometriosis is a condition where fragments of the lining of the uterus that is shed during menstruation embed outside the uterus, causing pain, scarring, infertility, and inflammation. Whereas the exact causes of endometriosis are not known, there is no clear evidence to show that inversions cause endometriosis. Physicians note that although the impact of yoga on the autonomic nervous system can affect menstrual flow, simply stretching and contracting tissues is unlikely to affect menstrual flow, which is not governed by gravity but by uterine contractions.

28. Is it safe to practice yoga after an injury?

Yoga is used not only to prevent injuries but also to promote recovery from a variety of injuries. Injury is largely prevented through yoga because the practice of asanas increases the range of motion at all joints and the length and strength in the musculature of the body in a balanced manner.

Injuries result from either accidents or through the habitual asymmetry we develop either in our normal course of living or in acquiring athletic or other occupational physical skills. Improper posture, repetitive motions, and overexertion of certain muscles and joints can lead to compression and tightening of muscles and joints, which in turn result in chronic pain.

Like any physical practice, it requires skill and knowledge to apply yoga to help heal a chronic or acute injury. So, if you are coming to yoga with an injury, the first order of business is to let your instructor know the details of your specific injury before you begin and at regular intervals as you delve into the practice. Yoga can indeed be beneficial in a number of injuries provided you proceed with caution and patience, work with an experienced teacher and follow your instructor's directions closely.

The most common injuries one suffers over a lifetime include sprains, strains and tears in the muscles, ligaments and tendons. Strains commonly occur in the lower back and hamstrings and are caused by overstretching a muscle or tendon. Sprains usually occur in ligaments that are connective tissues that connect two bones and are usually caused by a misaligned movement at the joint. Tears can accumulate in a muscle, ligament, or tendon over time and usually occurs through excessive load on a muscle so that it is extended beyond its biological capacity. Tears are commonly seen in the hamstrings, quadriceps, calves, and groins.

Rehabilitation using the aid of yoga asanas can be achieved, as per physicians and physical therapists, if you maintain caution and safety, establish stability and strength before creating mobility in the injured area, encourage rest and relaxation and practice patient self-restraint. For every type of injury, your instructor will let you know if you need to avoid certain poses or focus on others. For example, if the ACL, the anterior cruciate ligament that connects the thigh bone (femur) to the shin bone (tibia), is torn, it is recommended to avoid twisting the kneecap or meniscus as in pigeon pose or Baddha Konasana (bound angle pose). If the hamstrings have been overstretched, resulting in microtears in the muscle itself or at the tendons that join the three hamstrings to the back of the thigh bone, it is recommended to avoid deep forward-folding asanas and to keep the knees bent to reduce any strain on the hamstrings in milder forward-bending poses.

It is best to avoid fast-paced, flow-style yoga classes, including power yoga and Vinyasa classes after an injury. Instead, find a slow, alignment-based class that allows the use of props to help you attain the poses that are safe for you. Approach each pose with a sharp alertness toward the injured area and the rest of the body. Take stock of how you feel after each movement and ask your instructor how a pose can be modified to generate stability in the area of your injury.

Long-term immobilization of the affected area can lead to stiffness, loss of blood circulation, and even muscular and skeletal atrophy in the injured area. This is often seen when an arm has been in a cast for weeks, and the immobilized arms appears visibly thinner once the cast is removed. Yoga can help avoid such stiffness and atrophy if the movements can be performed safely and stably, after consulting your health care professional for any medical aid, such as bandages and other medical devices that promote stabilization of the injured area.

As a rule of thumb, during the initial or acute period of an initial, it is recommended to rest the injured area for four to six days, which includes not performing any movements that require strength in the injured area, that aggravate the injury, or that elicit pain. Because inflammation usually accompanies the acute stage of an injury, elevating the injured area through the judicious use of inversions can help control swelling and discomfort. Once the swelling has subsided, gentle yoga asanas can be performed to retain mobility, taking care not to stretch the muscles or trigger pain. During the subacute stages of an injury, in the two to three weeks following the week after the injury, very gentle stretching is recommended to begin rehabilitation, but this is to be done with a focus on the breath and sensation without stretching to the point where pain starts. Before creating mobility in the injured area, it is recommended to gently strengthen the muscles involved in the injury through slow, non-weight-bearing movements, being mindful to warm up and cool down before and after every session. Be mindful of any pain, tingling, or numbness during this phase, and seek medical advice if you find these symptoms arising. During the twelve to eighteen months following an injury—the chronic phase—the injured area remains highly susceptible to reinjury. It is recommended to not use excessive force during this phase of healing and continue to use yoga as a supplement to medical treatment and therapy.

29. What injuries are most likely to occur if yoga is done incorrectly?

Yoga students often encounter hamstring injuries, as do runners and athletes. However, whereas runners usually hurt the middle part or "belly" of the muscle at the center back of the thighs, in yoga, hamstring injury usually occurs just below the sit bones. The good news is that by learning the correct way to use the hamstrings, both athletes and yoga students can prevent and even heal hamstring injuries over time.

Injuries in yoga usually arise not because of a single event but from patterns and habits that we adopt largely unconsciously. Injuries therefore teach us by drawing our attention to harmful habitual patterns that would otherwise have slipped under the radar. Injuries, therefore, form a learning tool, teaching us new skills, such as patience, and increasing our awareness of our bodies and habits.

The hamstrings have two functions. One is to allow the knee to bend, as in walking or running. This action pulls us through our stride. When the lower end of the hamstring contracts, it allows the knee to bend and the lower leg to move backward.

The other function of the hamstrings is to hold us upright. This works the upper end of the hamstrings, where the muscle attaches to the sit bones. The hamstrings provide stability for the pelvis by drawing the sit bones toward the backs of the legs. This is what allows us to hold an erect posture.

Good posture develops when there is a balance between the muscle tones of the quadriceps at the front of the thighs and the hamstrings at the back of the thighs. Excessive practice or overexertion in either forward bends or backbends in yoga can hurt the hamstrings, throwing off the balance between the quadriceps and the hamstrings and, in certain cases, leading to tendinitis.

Tendons are strong connective tissue that attach muscles to bones. Over time, overstretching can cause tiny rips in the tendons that are initially felt as soreness but that in time can become very painful. In yoga, it is important to learn the right way to engage the muscles so that the tendons are not overtaxed. In a forward bend, it is therefore important to engage the hamstrings properly by engaging the top end of the hamstrings. You can feel the top end of the hamstring if while standing in a relaxed manner with your feet slightly separated and your knees slightly bent you pull back one foot without actually moving it back (isometric movement). This action makes the hamstrings pull the sit bones toward the knees.

To protect the upper end of the hamstring and the surrounding tendons, we must draw the sit bones toward the knees so that the hamstrings prevent overstretching in a forward bend, even while the muscle is lengthening (eccentric stretch). An eccentric stretch happens when the muscle remains engaged while it lengthens. For example, in Prasarita Padottanasana (wide-legged forward fold), this action would involve a downward drawing of the sit bones and hamstrings toward the knees, which would, in turn, create firmness in the area below the sit bones and a sense of stability in the hips.

Existing injuries in the upper end of the hamstring, below the sit bones, can be healed over time with a combination of relaxation, massage, and simple backbends. Dr. Ben Benjamin in Massage and Bodywork magazine suggests a simple massage technique that he calls "fractioning." This involves rubbing or plucking your finger across the length of the tendon in one direction with some pressure. Simple backbends such as Salabhasana (locust pose) and Chatushpadasana (bridge pose), practiced consistently while engaging the upper end of the hamstrings, will serve to strengthen the hamstrings.

30. Does greater flexibility lead to greater risk of injury?

Being inherently very flexible can put beginner yoga students at greater risk for injuries when they lack strength to support and stabilize the skeletal framework as the muscles extend and bend. The inflexible beginner in yoga is protected from overstretching and related injuries by the inherent tightness of the muscles.

Medically, extreme flexibility is called generalized joint hypermobility and can be both a genetic and acquired condition that increases the elasticity of connective tissues that hold our joints and organs together. Ehlers Danlos Syndrome is also accompanied by hypermobility but it is a more severe condition where patients suffer from severe joint and muscle pain, bruising, fatigue and are at increased risk of prolapses and hernias. Medical studies show that between 4 and 30 percent of the population have various degrees of hypermobility, although the it difficult to measure the true prevalence as there is no universal standard measure of flexibility. Moreover, flexibility varies with age, gender and race with older people, men and Caucasians being less flexible than younger people, women and non-Caucasians.

Although, increased elasticity and hyperflexibility can appear to be a good thing, it increases risk of injury because it means you now need to have more control around your joints to prevent them from hyperextending beyond their normal range. However, hyperflexibility affects not only the joints but also the tendons that hold bones together, ligaments that attach muscles to bones, and the muscles that are repeatedly extended beyond their capacity due to the excessive range at the joints. Hyperflexibility can lead to microtraumas in the skeletal framework and musculature, joint dislocations, and inflammation of the tendons and ligaments.

The primary issue is that most people are not aware of their hyperflexible condition in the first place. This is due to a general lack in body awareness and also partially due to a sedentary lifestyle. When such hyperflexible individuals take to certain physical activities such as dancing, gymnastics or yoga, the excessive flexibility is initially seen as an advantage and even encouraged until the student is injured. Moreover, when injured, hyperflexible individuals take longer to recover.

Yoga, when taught the right way, prevents hyperflexibility-related injuries because it cultivates awareness of alignment, increases our sensitivity of how the body is placed in space (proprioception) and builds strength before encouraging extension. This traditional, slow method of initiation into yoga can seem frustrating to the hyperflexible student who is constantly corrected in an alignment-based class to restrict the range of motion and pull back from deep extensions in forward and backward bends. However, this meticulous, time-consuming method of instruction builds strength and boosts neural feedback systems that provide information on how the joints, muscles, and other body parts are aligned in space and balance the extension and contraction of muscles with the mobility of the joints. In hyperflexible students, these neural feedback systems are impaired due to stretching beyond limits over time, further reducing control over the range of movement.

In some individuals, only certain joints, such as the shoulder joints or the hips or knees, are hypermobile and not the entire body. In such cases the muscles you need to strengthen will depend on which joints in your body are hypermobile. The key consideration is to develop the major muscles around the hypermobile joints and then learning to coordinate the muscles in the hypermobile region to work in coordination with the rest of the body.

The reason why yoga is beneficial for individuals with excessive flexibility is that it balances the building of strength in a coordinated manner with asanas that encourage extension of the joints, muscles, and connective tissues. The primary focus in yoga on cultivating the subtle sense of internal perception is also key in preventing injuries in hyperflexible students.

31. How do I know if I'm pushing myself too hard?

It is the current culture globally, but particularly in the West, to push ourselves beyond our limits to achieve our goals. Phrases like "work harder," "whatever it takes," "push through it," and "go that extra mile" are common parlance in our work and sports. This attitude has resulted in widespread stress and anxiety in people from all walks of life and established a culture based on external parameters of success and competitiveness.

However, yoga is based on an ancient philosophy that discourages such a mindset. The Yoga Sutras, the first compiled text on yoga by Patanjali, talks about a balance of effort and ease in all yoga poses. One of the primary reasons for injury in yoga is pushing yourself too hard and trying an asana when your body is not ready for it. Exerting excessive effort in achieving what we have set as our goal is so ingrained in us that we find it hard to approach yoga in the light of its underlying philosophy. But practicing yoga with a sole focus on its third limb of physical asanas is not only superficial but also dangerous.

One of the primary dangers—adopting only the physical aspects of yoga with no understanding of its philosophy—is due to our socially and culturally conditioned nature of pushing ourselves too hard to achieve. This attitude, more often than not, results in injury that leads students to abandon the practice of yoga altogether.

On the other extreme, some of us are overly cautious and don't push ourselves enough. Continuously holding ourselves back keeps us in our comfort zone, stunts our potential and dulls both the body and mind over time.

Yoga encourages mindfully going up to the edge of your abilities and exploring your mental and physical capabilities in a skilled manner. Yoga is often defined as skillful action—not only on the mat but in our day-to-day lives as well. The first phase of yoga (yamas) begins with the tenet of nonviolence (ahimsa), as popularly known from the speeches and activism of Mahatma Gandhi. Nonviolence implies compassion and kindness toward yourself as well. By pushing ourselves too hard, or not at all, we are being unkind to ourselves. This initial phase of yoga also teaches contentment and acceptance (santosha). It is only in accepting what and who we are in the present moment that we can hope to build on it.

The challenge in developing and maintaining a life-long yoga practice, is to approach each practice session with a beginner's mind. This means being highly observant of your mind and body as you are in the present moment. The aim is not to develop a static routine or yoga sequence that you practice every day. The aim is to use the asanas and the focus on the breath as tools to refining your capacities of observation, self-examination and analysis. You instinctively know when you are pushing yourself too hard. Your body lets you know through pain and injuries. You also intuitively know when you are holding back and erring on the side of caution and comfort. Your body lets you know through the lack of progress, stagnation, dullness, boredom, and even deterioration over time. So, keep a beginner's mind that is open to possibilities. Neither push yourself too hard nor hold back, but explore your edge and in time you will find your edge has shifted toward new horizons.

How to Practice Yoga

32. How do I know what type of yoga is best for me?

As a brief search online will show you, there are many styles and schools of yoga. Although all yoga is based on the same philosophy, the different schools adopt either slight variations of traditional styles or adopt a specific focus for branding. Depending for what you are looking for in yoga, carefully trying out different forms and teachers while mindfully observing how your body, mind, and spirit react to the practice, the teacher, and the environment will be the key to finding what type of yoga is best for you. When you do decide to try a particular school, it is advisable that you try one school and one teacher at a time instead of attending several yoga classes in a short span of time. The effects of any form and style of yoga on the body take time to manifest and patience and a keen skill of observation to notice. Therefore, when you do decide to try out a yoga class, give it at least three to six months to accurately gauge the effect it has on your body. After this initial trial period, you could decide whether to keep going to the same class or try out another.

Traditional styles include schools like the Shivananda school of yoga, the Iyengar school of yoga, Kundalini yoga, and so on. All traditional schools of yoga acknowledge and are deeply respectful of their lineage of usually a long line of yoga teachers down the ages, and they ultimately attribute their practice to the teachings of Patanjali. If you're looking for a spiritual, supportive yoga community and are seeking answers to deeper questions in addition to a physical practice, these traditional schools of yoga might be worth attending.

Modern schools of yoga tend to place more emphasis on the scientific basis of their practice and develop special sequences and environments in which they must be practiced. For example, the popular hot yoga is practiced in heated rooms and adopts a restricted sequence of twenty-six poses that are practiced in a cyclical fashion. This form of yoga has been scientifically established to improve cardiovascular health and lose weight. So, if you're looking for a high-energy form of yoga with the aim of losing or maintaining weight or increasing cardiac health, attending classes such as hot yoga or power yoga or a Vinyasa ashtanga flow yoga class might be the forms you're looking for. Such energetic classes are also ideally suited for different kinds of athletes.

On the other hand, if your goal is to practice yoga to recover from an injury or a surgery or some other physical or mental ailment, it is advisable to seek one-on-one help in a private yoga class or, better still, in a yoga therapy session. Whereas all yoga offer therapeutic benefits and private sessions allow for a practice targeted at the student's current concerns, yoga therapists are particularly trained for this approach. Yoga therapists are trained not only to teach yoga in such a way that the student benefits physically and psychologically from the session but also to teach with the physical or mental issue that the student is currently dealing with, front and center.

If you are looking for deep relaxation from a hectic, busy life, on the other hand, you might want to opt for a class that has a slower pace and holds each pose for a sustained length of time. Yin yoga and Restorative yoga classes are specifically designed for deep relaxation. Iyengar yoga classes, although focused on alignment, also used props and include restorative sessions.

Just as important as finding the type of yoga that is right for you is finding the teacher who is best for you. Finding a suitable teacher is not a task to be taken lightly. This is because the student needs to have a deep sense of respect and trust in the teacher. This is not an easy thing to do in this day and age. Respect is a necessity in the physical and spiritual path and practice of yoga, not simply because of the traditional conventions of yoga but also because without respect it is difficult and almost impossible to attune yourself to the subtlety of the teachings and thereby to learn what is being taught.

Trust is necessary in the physical and spiritual paths of yoga because as a student, one is by definition ignorant of the subject and one needs to trust that the teacher is taking you on the right path. More so in the modern day than perhaps in ancient times, we are surrounded by a constant sense of fear. In the Western world, our sense of individuality and personal space makes us wary or physical touch. In learning yoga, the student must be able to let go of such fears because yoga involves understanding your boundaries and pushing forward. Moreover, in many traditional and modern schools of yoga, the teacher physically adjusts the student to teach correct posture, alignment, and balance in an asana. If the student cannot trust the teacher with such close contact, both psychologically and physically, it can lead to different kinds of problems.

33. How do I know I'm ready for pranayama practice?

Pranayama is the practice of rechanneling bioenergy in the body through the mindful control of breathing. It is a subtle and intense practice. Traditionally, the body is trained for strength, flexibility, physical endurance, and mental stability through the practice of yoga postures or asanas for at least a few years before the student is introduced to the practice of pranayama.

Daily life is full of engrossing distractions. As such, it is difficult to draw the mind inward and pay close attention to the movement of breath and its effects on the body. Therefore, it is important to develop a regular practice of asanas so that the mind is trained to pay attention to subtle changes in the body before one attempts pranayama.

Some schools of yoga have definite requirements for introduction into pranayama practice. For example, in the Mysore style of Ashtanga yoga, spearheaded by Pattabhi Jois, students are required to successfully complete the third series of asanas before starting pranayama. In the Iyengar school of yoga, students need to be at least established in a regular level I practice before starting pranayama. In the Sivananda school of yoga, pranayama can be introduced into daily practice together with asanas.

One of the main reasons a steady, comfortable practice of asanas is encouraged before one starts practicing pranayama is that pranayama requires the practitioner to sit in a meditative posture for extended periods. Sitting completely still is not an easy task, physically or mentally. The practice of asanas helps us develop the skill of sitting still for long periods. This requires open hips, strong arms, an expansive chest, and the ability to remain still and alert.

Open hips are brought about by standing poses, particularly where the legs are wide apart or pulled behind the torso. Strong arms are brought about by poses that balance the weight of the body partially or completely on the arms. An expansive, open chest is developed through the practice of deep backbends. And an ability to remain still and alert is brought about by holding challenging poses for extended periods.

In addition to the musculoskeletal structure of the body, the internal organs are massaged, expanded or contracted during the practice of kumbhakas and bandhas that are an integral part of the practice of pranayama. Beginning the practice of kumbhakas and bandhas requires a steady and regular practice of asanas, so that the internal organs and various functional systems of the body develop the resilience and strength to withstand the practice.

The word "kumbhaka" means "pot" in Sanskrit. In the practice of kumbhakas in pranayama, the torso is considered a pot with two openings— Tone at the mouth and one at the base of the pelvis. Kumbhakas denote the retention of breath and can be of two types. One can hold the breathing cycle either after breathing in (antara kumbhaka) or after breathing out (bahya kumbhaka). Biological breath retention increases the levels of carbon dioxide and carbonic acid in the blood. Slight increases in the levels of carbon dioxide and carbonic acid in the blood has several biological benefits. It dilates blood vessels bringing more blood into your brain and heart. It dilates the passages of the lungs (bronchi) and allows more air to enter your lungs in the following cycles. It calms the nervous system and reduces your need and craving for food, particularly food high in acid content.

Bandhas are energetic locks and are of four main types. Mula bandha or the root lock is the locking of energy at the base of the pelvis and is accompanied by drawing the floor of the pelvis including the rectal wall up and into the body. Jalandhara bandha or throat lock, locks energy at the nerves and vessels in the neck area. Uddiyana bandha is a diaphragmatic lock. The diaphragm is the dome shaped muscle that separates the abdomen from the thoracic cavity. Uddiyana bandha is accompanied by a lift of the diaphragm and a false inhalation, that is, all the actions of breathing in without actually allowing air into your lungs. Maha bandha or the ultimate energetic lock occurs when all three locks are engaged simultaneously.

Mr. Iyengar himself had been advised by his teacher, Krishnamacharya, that he was not ready for the practice of Pranayama. However, Iyengar spied on his teacher and started practicing on his own. Although it is true, that a certain level of physical skill and endurance are needed to prevent injuries in the path of Pranayama, a lot is learnt through trial and error.

34. Should I learn yoga from a book, an online course, a group class, or a private class?

A book on yoga can offer a detailed and exhaustive source of information on yoga postures (asanas), the importance of the different stages on yoga as well as the philosophy on which the practice of yoga is based. Although books on yoga, such as this, offer you theoretical knowledge on yoga, and yoga books with images can be an engrossing launchpad to try out some yoga poses, it is not where you would necessarily go to develop your practical knowledge of yoga and a personal practice.

Online courses on yoga come in different shapes and forms. They can be lectures—both audio and video—or demonstrations of yoga poses. They can also be interactive where your questions are answered either on an online discussion forum or on a one-on-one video conference. Technology is improving at an incredible rate. It is possible to gain the benefits of a one-on-one class from an online course, provided you and your teacher have access to the right technology and are willing to experiment with teaching and learning protocols that are amenable to communication via video.

Given that the field of online courses on yoga is still highly experimental, it does have some distinct disadvantages. First, during a class where the teacher is physically present with the student, be it in a group class or an individual class, the teacher is able to view the student from an entire 360-degree vantage point along all dimensions. This allows the teacher to pinpoint and identify errors and adjustments in real time. Perhaps with the advancement of technology, online courses on yoga can only be hooked up to three dimensional cameras. But as of now, this is not commonplace, and therefore online classes restrict the ability of the teacher to identify and offer corrections and make hands-on adjustments impossible.

Advantages of online courses include a greater degree of structure to the classes, possibly better visibility of the teacher compared to a group class, the ability to download entire class sequences and play them over and over again like a chess game to improve your practice, as well as access to online discussion forums that offer you a sense of community with your teacher and fellow students where you can ask and clarify your doubts at your own pace and level of comfort.

Groups classes have several advantages and disadvantages over both online courses and private classes. The size of the group class matters as well. Large group classes generate a sense of energy that permeates throughout the students and teacher. This elevates your practice in subconscious ways, allowing you to put in more than you could have in a private practice or a small group class. Group yoga classes allow the teacher to use students as models to emphasize a teaching point that might otherwise not be conveyed. This allows students who learn better visually to understand the point being taught. Group classes also allow students to learn from each other's mistakes and develop a sense of direct community that is different from the undeniable distance in virtual communities. Moreover, students are often partnered up in both large and small classes where one student acts as a prop or facilitator of another student. This allows students to help each other in their personal journey and offers a benefit not available in online or private classes.

Traditionally, yoga was taught largely in private sessions between the teacher (guru) and student (shishya). This tradition is called the guru-shishya parampara. There are several advantages to long-term, one-on-one private classes with a single teacher. Undoubtedly, private classes offer a personal touch where the teacher's entire attention is focused solely on you and the class is tailored to your specific needs and requests. Students generally opt for a private yoga class when they are trying yoga for the first time, when they are looking for answers to personal questions, when they prefer a greater level of guidance, when they need or want personal attention to improve or recover from an injury, when they want to learn more about the philosophy, when they want to relax or meditate, when they want to focus on specific poses, or when they want to feel more confident before they attend a group class.

The disadvantage of a private yoga class is that it puts both the student and teacher in a more vulnerable position. This can be remedied by conducting detailed research on your teacher before making a choice. Even for students who have been attending private yoga sessions with a particular teacher for a long time, it can be an intimidating experience as you have the teacher's attention on you the whole time and cannot get lost in the crowd. For some, this is an advantage, but for others, it can also be intimidating and stressful.

Based on this discussion, your choice of classes or courses on yoga will depend on your specific needs are inclinations. If you enjoy social learning, you might try out a group class. If you enjoy a one-on-one focused and intense approach, you might try out a private class. If you are not looking to practice yoga but simply want information on it, you might want to pick up a book on yoga. Whatever your choice, put some thought into it, and if you find your initial choices do not suit you, do not hesitate to change them.

35. What should I look for in a yoga teacher?

An ancient Indian proverb says, "When the student is ready, the teacher appears." This finding of the ideal teacher usually involves an extensive, intensive search and some good luck on the part of the student.

With a multitude of yoga studios cropping up like wildflowers, it can be difficult to know how to find the yoga teacher right for you. Taking a multipronged approach can help you find the teacher ideal for you.

First and foremost, hone and trust your gut instincts. This is important in any decision-making process, but particularly in the case of finding a yoga teacher. After taking a few classes with a yoga teacher, pay careful attention to whether what is being taught and the way it is being taught is indeed the direction you want to go. Do not worry about whether you fit in, in terms of current skills or abilities, because these will change over time with practice. Although decisions made in the blink of an eye may not always be correct, trusting your gut goes a long way in finding the best yoga teacher for you.

In your initial classes, you must observe your teacher intently. If you are looking to develop a meditative practice with a focus on alignment, is this what your teacher is doing in class? Or is the teacher more likely to teacher a power yoga class? Match your needs to the content of the teacher's class. It is beneficial to attend classes with the same teacher over an extended period. However, this can only prove beneficial if your learning goals match the teacher's teaching interests.

In addition to observing your teacher, you must also observe the effect the teacher has on you. For example, sometimes a teacher can appear overly strict or critical. In other words, being in the presence of this teacher might take you out of your comfort zone. But the enduring effect of this teacher on you might be to propel you toward improving rapidly. In such cases you might realize that the teacher's strict, critical approach is simply his or her personal style of delivery and is not in conflict with your betterment. At other times, a teacher can be sweet and lenient, being careful to consider your zone of comfort and sensitive to your boundaries. However, you may find you are making no progress under this teacher's guidance. In such a case you might want to keep searching for your ideal teacher who not only caters to your inherent sensibilities but also shows you the direction toward progress.

Some students come to yoga with a predetermined decision of making a career as a yoga teacher. Although this is not ideal, if you know this is what you intend, you will need to find a yoga teacher who can help guide you to acquire the requisite credentials to become a yoga teacher. In the United States, this means you will need to find out whether your teacher is certified by the Yoga Alliance® as a Registered Yoga Teacher®. Do not hesitate to ask your teachers where they studied, with whom, and for how long. In fact, note whether your teacher is approachable and answers your questions with care. You should always prefer those yoga teachers who are lifelong students themselves and continue to further their own education in yoga by attending regular yoga workshops and learning under more experienced teachers.

36. How do I begin, maintain, and grow my yoga practice?

The renowned yoga teacher B.K.S. Iyengar is known to have said, "In the beginning to set things in motion, there is no substitute for sweat."

As with everything, beginning your yoga practice is always the most difficult part. Knowing and reminding yourself regularly of why you are taking up the practice of yoga can not only help you determine what type or style of yoga is ideal for you (as discussed earlier) but will also help you adhere to your practice with determination and regularity. Students come to yoga for different reasons: for physical strength and flexibility, to combat mental stress and maintain emotional equilibrium, and for spiritual growth. Know the reasons that brought you to yoga. In fact, maintain a written journal of your reasons for practicing, the contents and components of your practice, and the effects that you observe in yourself.

In the beginning, as well as throughout your growth in yoga, talk to more experienced students and teachers. You will find that everyone struggled to start their personal yoga practice, and everyone continues to struggle as their lives go through their own rhythms of ups and downs.

To overcome the initial hurdles and inertia in launching your yoga practice, a simple and yet highly effective strategy is to predetermine when, where, and for how long you'll be practicing your yoga and set up your practice space. Even though it may not be possible for you to have a dedicated space for your practice, it is helpful to organize your available living space to include an area for your yoga practice. If you intend to practice early in the morning, it is a good idea to lay out your yoga mat and any props you want to use, such as a strap, yoga blocks, blankets, and bolsters, the night before.

Putting some thought into getting or choosing comfortable clothes and making dietary adjustments might also help in overcoming some of the obstacles in beginning your yoga practice. Students prefer wearing leggings or shorts and a top of a breathable material, preferably cotton, during practice. Although stretchable leggings are flexible and attractive, shorts are preferable, as they do not hinder poses where the friction from skin-to-skin contact is helpful and even necessary, such as tree pose (Vrykshasana) or arm balances such as the crane pose (Bakasana).

Finding the right kind of diet and eating schedule that fosters your yoga practice might need some trial and error. The idea is to balance the content and quantity of your diet such that you have adequate energy for your practice but are not actively digesting your meal or feeling hungry during your practice. For most students, eating something light containing slow-digesting carbohydrates and fiber, such as oatmeal, grains, fruits, and vegetables, a few hours before your practice works best. Staying hydrated is also key in preventing muscle cramps and promoting flexibility during your practice.

Once you have started practicing yoga daily at a fixed time during the day, you will notice that your practice waxes and wanes as life progresses. There are some days when you will feel you have made considerable progress, days when you will be trying to simply hold on to what you have learned, and other days when you will feel you're backtracking. To maintain your yoga practice through it all, you need to arrive on your yoga mat every day and do your best, irrespective of how you feel about it. Progress will only be discernible with continuous, long-term practice.

To grow and develop your personal yoga practice, learning continuously is key. Attend yoga classes regularly, read books on yoga and write in your yoga journal. Include meditation and breathing practices that show you the path to making progress, not only physically but also mentally and spiritually. In keeping your spirits up during the upheavals of personal growth, it is helpful to be part of a yoga community or a group of yoga students who are willing to discuss their own journeys. Discussing your questions and concerns with each other can reveal unexpected solutions.

37. How frequently should I practice yoga or take classes?

You should practice yoga every day. Even practicing yoga up to three to five times a day is encouraged. Incremental benefits such as increased energy, mobility, and flexibility can be seen only when you practice regularly.

However, yoga classes are where you generally learn yoga but do not necessarily practice yoga. There is an important distinction between learning and practicing yoga. It is true that when you learn a new asana, it is advisable to include it in your practice in the days following your class so that you can understand its intricacies and assimilate the teachings. However, your body may not be ready for all that you happen to be taught in a class. In such cases it is advisable to use props and practice preparatory poses first, during your daily home practice, rather than attempt an asana or pranayama that is too difficult for you.

An important idea to consider when practicing yoga daily is "playing the edge." This refers to the need to push yourself to the edge of your abilities without crossing the limits of your capacity. This is only possible when students goes slow and pays close attention to their body, mind, and spirit during and after their yoga practice.

When practicing yoga every day or multiple times a day, it is also important to switch up your routine or yoga sequence and not repeat the same sequence every day. There are two important reasons behind adopting new sequences in your daily practice.

First, it prevents injuries that arise out of repetition. Particularly when we are beginners, the likelihood of making errors in practicing a particular asana or pranayama is high. If these errors are repeated frequently, the chances of injury increase. It is therefore judicious to practice a posture or breath mindfully, paying close attention to the positive and negative effects on your body, mind, and spirit and place these questions before your teacher in the following class. This means that at the beginner level, it is a good idea to take classes at least once or twice a week so you can get your doubts clarified before your body gets subconsciously set in an incorrect method of practicing a posture or breathing technique.

Second, many schools of yoga and experienced teachers believe repeating the same sequence again and again, without careful thought, reduces your capacity to approach an asana with a beginner's mind. The idea is that the approach and attitude with which you practice yoga is just as important as what you are practicing. If you repeat the same sequence every day, thoughtlessly, it is not yoga. Therefore, it is important to analyze your practice every day and design your practice based on the knowledge you have obtained in class while at the same time listening to your own body and respecting its needs and limitations.

The frequency with which you attend classes depends on your accessibility to yoga classes. At present, yoga classes are also available online, and it is possible to take such classes without the restrictions of commuting. However, if you want to attend classes in person and are unable to do so, it is also possible to benefit from occasional workshops and classes with expert teachers, provided you develop your own daily practice routine at home.

38. What should I wear to yoga class?

The most important considerations for yoga class clothing are comfort, allowing your teacher to view the alignment of your body, and modesty.

This means you would want to wear clothes that allow you to move in them without straining your bones and muscles or overly stretching your skin. Some fabrics such as polyester, nylon, and spandex stretch to a great extent but are not breathable materials. On the other hand, purely natural fabrics like linen and cotton are breathable but not flexible. You will find an array of yoga wear in sporting stores and online that combine different materials to allow comfort, flexibility and breathability.

Breathable material that wicks moisture prevents or reduces the growth of bacteria on the skin. During yoga, particularly when you are a beginner, you tend to sweat profusely. Breathable, moisture-wicking material allows you to remain cool and dry throughout your practice or class. This is particularly important during the humid summer months. Breathable, flexible material allows air to flow in and out without flopping on your skin in baggy creases. The fabric prevents your body from overheating so that you don't feel stuffy and uncomfortable.

Allowing your teacher to easily visualize the alignment of your body is also an important consideration while choosing yoga clothes. Baggy clothes like sweatpants or buddha pants may be very comfortable and airy and allow you to move in them but they cover the alignment of your knees and ankles. This prevents your yoga teacher from ascertaining whether your body is in the right alignment and offering valuable feedback.

Another important consideration for more advanced students who regularly practice inversions is that you would not want your clothes to ride up when you are in an inversion. This is a tricky requirement. One way to prevent clothes from riding up during inversions is to wear leotards as in dance or gymnastic attire. However, leotards are not convenient for yoga poses that require skin-to-skin contact for stability or balance. In such cases, wearing a top that tucks into shorts or pants prevents clothes from riding up during inversions.

Perhaps less important but of practical importance is the durability and economy of your yoga clothing. Commercially available yoga clothes are generally made to be durable so that they last a long time before they need to be replaced, making them economical. Fabric with some percentage of Spandex or Elastane increases flexibility and durability.

When buying yoga wear made of composite fabrics, materials to look out for are bamboo, nylon, Spandex, cotton, and polyester. Bamboo is light, soft, breathable, and moisture-wicking. Nylon dries quickly and is soft. Clothing with around 75–80 percent nylon is breathable and moisture wicking as well. Spandex, also known as Lycra or elastane, has exceptional elasticity, and offers comfort and flexibility. Cotton is natural and breathable, but it absorbs moisture, wrinkles easily, and takes a long time to dry. However, when combined with synthetic materials such as spandex, it increases the natural feel. Polyester is durable, lightweight, breathable, and wrinkle-resistant. If you intend to practice yoga outdoors, polyester and bamboo also protect you against the ultraviolet rays of the sun.

Modesty in day-to-day wear does not appear to be as important of a concern in Western societies as it is in the East. However, considering that the practice of yoga originated in the East, and it is essentially a spiritual practice, you might want to consider wearing modestly designed apparel at yoga classes. This is not only respectful but will also allow you to focus more on your practice than on external elements. This means, for example, that if you are a woman, you would want to stay away from low-cut tops, and if you are a man, you would want to avoid floppy shorts. Also, remember, your choice of apparel should be such that it stays in place even during inversions.

39. What should I eat to aid my yoga practice?

Food fads come and go. There are no specific restrictions and no strict diet regimens for the student of yoga. However, in keeping with the basic tenet of ahimsa (meaning nonharming or nonviolence), dedicated and serious students of yoga generally do not eat meat, fish, or eggs, although most do consume milk and milk products, particularly if they follow Ayurvedic guidelines. Ayurveda is a sister discipline of yoga and also developed in ancient India.

The most important thing to note is that what you eat in twelve to twenty-four hours preceding your yoga practice determines how your body reacts to it. It is advisable to not eat in the two to three hours before a yoga session. However, starving for long periods before a yoga session is also discouraged. A light, simple, plant-based diet taken at regular times, two to three hours before a practice session, prevents fatigue, energizes the body and mind, and stimulates your inherent life force (prana).

Experts in yoga and Ayurveda recommend staying away, and preferably eliminating, caffeine, alcohol, tobacco, refined sugar, artificial chemicals, and genetically modified foods. Yoga is all about moderation, so eating something that you would rather avoid is okay once in a while, but it is important to make the choice consciously and note the effect it has on your body, mind, and, above all, your practice.

Counterintuitively, yoga discourages using your willpower to actively avoid any food, or anything for that matter. This is because active avoidance using will power, as per yoga philosophy, develops a desire, even if it is a desire to avoid. And all forms of desire, positive or negative, are obstacles in the practice of yoga. Therefore, instead of actively wanting or avoiding certain foods, it is more important to pay close attention to how you feel during your yoga practice after having consumed a particular food (Svadhyaya or self-study). In time, as your practice develops, you will organically adopt a diet that allows your body to feel at ease during your yoga practice.

After you have eaten, notice whether it makes you feel energetic or whether it makes you feel like taking a nap. If you feel drowsy after a meal, it means it is taking up energy rather than providing energy for you. Notice whether your mind feels dull or sharp after a meal. This tells you how your nervous system reacts to the food you have just eaten. Also notice itching of the skin and a raised heartbeat after a meal, as these may be signs of being allergic to a food item you've consumed.

Ayurveda determines ideal food groups for individuals based on their constitution. According to Ayurveda, body constitutions (Sanskrit, Doshas) comprise broadly three types or combinations thereof. These three constitutions are vata, kapha, and pitta. (Please refer to Question 23 for details on the characteristics of the three types of constitutions). Generally, people of vata constitution are encouraged to eat root vegetables, such as yams, beets, potatoes, radishes, parsnips, turnips, rutabagas, carrots, yuca, kohlrabi, onions, garlic, turmeric, ginger, and so on. Root vegetables have a grounding effect on the airy vata constitution. People of pitta constitution are encouraged to eat salads and milk products. These have a cooling, soothing effect on the fiery pitta constitution. People of kapha constitution are encouraged to eat spicy, tangy foods such as chilies and tomatoes. These have a heating effect on the overly grounded kapha constitution.

40. How should I sequence yoga poses in my practice?

Remarkably, the order in which you practice yoga postures changes the effect the practice session has on your body. Learning to sequence effectively plays an important role in developing a yoga practice suited to your unique needs and body type. Sequencing of yoga poses can either have an energizing or calming effect on your body after the session is over. The advantage of knowing how to sequence your practice can help you manage symptoms of hyperstimulation, restlessness, depression, stress or anxiety.

There are different ways of sequencing yoga sessions. One of the ways to view sequencing of yoga poses is to view asanas as part of larger categories. The most common broad categories of postures are standing poses, forward bends, backbends, inversion, arm balances, and twists. These categories are overlapping. For example, Adho Mukha Vrykshasana (handstand) is an arm balance and an inversion; Uttanasana (intense forward fold) is both a standing pose and a forward bend.

Each of the different categories of yoga postures have distinct and unmistakable energetic effects on the body. Asanas that extend the spine backward such as Urdhva Dhanurasana (upward bow pose) are stimulating. Most inversions and standing poses are stimulating and energizing as well, though less so than poses where the spine bends backward. On the other hand, as you might expect, asanas where the spine extends forward, such as Paschimottanasana (intense westward stretch), are relaxing. Generally increasing the duration of holding forward or backward bends or increasing the intensity of the internal extension of the spine increases the relaxing or stimulating effect of the asana. Asanas where the spine twists, such as Parivritta Trikonasana (revolved triangle pose), have a balancing and cleansing effect on the body.

Therefore, one way to sequence your practice is to focus a sequence on a particular category, increasing the level of difficulty as the sequence progresses. For example, a beginner level sequence focused on forward bends might start with Uttanasana (intense forward fold), progress through Parshvottanasana (intense side stretch), Prasarita Padottanasana (widelegged forward fold), and Janu Sirsasana (head to knee forward bend), and work its way up to Paschimottanasana (intense westward stretch). As the difficulty level of your sequences increases you might incorporate progressively more difficult forward bends in your sequence such as Malasana (garland pose) and Kurmasana (tortoise pose).

Similarly, other sequences practice could incorporate solely standing poses, backbends, arm balances or twists. Although such sequencing is entirely possible, commonly practiced and promotes a deep and focused practice, there are some poses you might want to incorporate more frequently in your practice, irrespective of what category of asanas you are focusing on in a particular sequence. For example, Adho Mukha Shvanasana is an important asana in most schools and styles of yoga. It not only extends the spine, but also stretches the legs and strengthens the arms. This pose in itself includes elements of all categories of asanas except twists.

Similarly, whatever group of asanas a specific practice sequence is focused on, you would always want to incorporate some inversions in your sequence, unless there is a specific physical incapacity to do so. Although, there is no specific point in your sequence where you must introduce inversions, once you are capable of doing both, Sirsasana (headstand) should always be done before Sarvangasana (shoulder stand).

Another way to sequence a yoga session is to aim for balance. This implies balancing energizing and stimulating asanas with calming and relaxing asanas. Twists are in themselves balancing. In addition, you can promote balance by countering forward bending poses with backward bending poses. This must be done judiciously and in moderation, however, as frequent alternation of forward and backward bends can be detrimental for the spine.

The options to skillfully sequencing your yoga sessions are limitless. Sequences can be linear, that is, progressing from less challenging poses to more challenging poses. Sequences can be cyclical where a given set of poses is repeated with or without slight variations. Sequences can have a peak, where all preceding poses are sequenced to facilitate and prepare you for different components of the peak pose followed by a short or prolonged cooling down phase. Sequences may be designed around a particular goal or benefit such as alleviating backpain, shoulder stiffness, migraines or depression.

Although there are no set patterns to how you will start or progress through your yoga sequence, every yoga session generally culminates in Shavasana or the corpse pose. Shavasana, apparently the simplest, and in reality the most difficult of all asanas, is the conscious, alert, and active letting go of all sensations and fluctuations of the mind. Ending your yoga sessions with Shavasana allows you to internalize the effects of your practice and realigns your body and mind to face the world.

If you would like to know more about how to sequence your yoga practice, you will find details about a book on yoga sequencing in the bibliography at the end of this book.

41. What types of hands-on assists should I expect from my teacher in yoga class?

In a yoga class, it is often expected that your teacher will be giving you hands-on assists. This can range from light touches to indicate an anatomical point that you should focus on as you are trying to master an asana, to forceful movements that move you into an asana. Hands-on assists can help find better alignment. They can help you relax into a pose. They can help you find stability. Or they can guide your attention to anatomical points or lines of energy.

Touch, unlike verbal instruction, is more direct and intimate, and can be easily misunderstood. In the West, it is customary for teachers to ask for the student's consent before offering hands-on assists. This allows students to either accept the assist or refuse it if they find it uncomfortable. For more on this topic, see the following question.

One of the poses that you could expect a hands-on assist in is Tadasana (mountain pose) as well as in most standing poses. In standing poses, it is difficult to distribute your weight evenly across to the weight-bearing points of the sole of your feet. Many tend to place most of their body weight on the insides of their feet, causing their arches to flatten (pronation), while many others place most of their body weight on the outer edges of their feet causing the inner arches to rise or tilt outward (supination). In order to bring attention to this disbalance, you may expect your yoga teachers to place their hands on the tops of your feet and apply pressure on either the inner or outer edges to help you distribute your body weight more evenly.

Balancing poses are another group of poses where hands-on assists can be very helpful. Often, even with adequate strength and flexibility, we find it difficult to find our balance in poses such as Virabhadrasana III (warrior pose III). Teachers may choose to offer hands-on assists in warrior pose III by lightly connecting their hip to the outer hip of the standing leg and touching the heel of the extended leg with one hand and the top of the upper shoulders with the other hand. This gives proprioceptive awareness to the students of where their leg and torso are in space, helping them to find greater extension and balance.

Balance is also crucial in inversions such as Sirsasana (headstand) and Pincha Mayurasana (forearm balance). Students generally start off at the wall, in the case of inversions. However, soon students grow dependent on the wall and find it difficult to practice inversions in the center of the room. Fear plays a major role in attempting to balance without any support in sight. In such scenarios, hands-on assists can help students connect with their foundation and gain more control while upside down. In the case of forearm balance, teachers usually stand behind the student and place their feet gently on the student's hands and wrists. This brings awareness to the surface of the palms and forearms that are in contact with the ground. Teachers may also support the hips on either side or place a fist between the student's calves. This helps bring attention to the center line of the body, maintaining balance.

Sometimes, if used intelligently, hands-on assists can prevent injuries in overenthusiastic students. For example, students who exert excessive effort, particularly students who are hyperflexible, can often injure their hamstrings in forward-folding asanas. The hands-on assists in these forward-folding poses prevent students from going too deep into the pose with a view to preventing injury. For example, in Prasarita Padottanasana (wide-legged forward fold), the teachers place their hands on either side of the hips and apply pressure backward and downward. This prevents the sacrum and hip girdle from over-rotating forward and stabilizes the hamstrings, preventing injury.

42. How do I respond to hands-on adjustments in a yoga class?

Yoga teachers, both in ancient and modern times, in India, the United States, and the world over, have provided hands-on guidance to their disciples and students.

The advantages of subtle or energetic hands-on assists can be profound. It can help students move deeper into the asana and move beyond what they had thought they were capable of. An intelligent hands-on assist is as direct as learning can get. Yoga involves subtle skill. This skill cannot be completely conveyed in words. Demonstrations help, but subtle movements and energetic alignments are difficult to demonstrate. Even when an asana is skillfully demonstrated by the teacher, students might not grasp the subtleties of the movement or the action, or pinpoint the origin and progression of the movement or flow of energy in their own bodies. In such cases, skillful and intelligent hands-on assists are illuminating.

However, many teachers are now steering away from hands-on assists for a number of reasons. First, unless the teacher is highly skilled and attentive of the student's needs, energetic alignment based hands-on assists can be potentially dangerous and can lead to injury. Some assists can push students past the limitations of their capacities. These types of injuries stem from overambitious hands-on assists and can be avoided with increased skill, intelligence, and patience on the part of the teacher, as well as limitations and boundaries being stated clearly on the part of the student.

The wide circulation of images of difficult yoga poses has fetishized extreme flexibility, particularly in the context of yoga. This, against the backdrop of an inherent social culture in the West that glorifies competition, quick results, and maximum effort, leads undertrained teachers to prematurely push students more deeply into an asana than they are ready for. A high level of training needs to be instated before a teacher is capable of providing hands-on assists. On the other hand, a student should feel comfortable in refusing hands-on assists at any point without being or appearing disrespectful. Setting an atmosphere where the student is comfortable in opting out of receiving hands-on assists is largely dependent on the teacher.

Some teachers offer the use of cards to indicate whether the student is open to receiving hands-on assists or not. This has the advantage of not only being discreet but allowing students to change their minds during class by simply flipping the card.

Second, we live in an increasingly litigious society. Recent global incidents of sexual harassment in yoga classes have brought heightened awareness to the power dynamics in a yoga class. On one hand, students naturally crave the attention and affection of their teachers, and on the other, teachers have at times been incapable of maintaining their perspective and boundaries. These tendencies have led to complications in both giving and receiving hands-on assists in yoga classes.

Overall, you will need to decide on how you want to respond to hands-on assists. Your choice of yoga class and teacher will determine the level of hands-on assists you might expect. For example, in a fast-paced flow yoga class, where the teacher demonstrates the poses as the students follow along, will have little opportunity for hands-on assists, whereas an alignment-based yoga class focuses on perfecting subtle movements and can incorporate hands-on assists in a variety of asanas.

43. How can I get more comfortable sitting cross-legged? Can I still do yoga if I cannot sit cross-legged?

Sukhasana, or the "easy pose" where you sit cross-legged, may not be easy at all, particularly if you have tight hamstrings. In Sukhasana, the shins are crossed such that the feet can be tucked under the creases of the knees when sitting.

The more advanced asana in sitting cross-legged is Padmasana, or lotus pose. Here, instead of crossing the shins and tucking the feet under the knees, the feet rest on top of the opposite thighs with the soles of the feet turned upward. When the legs cross loosely, it is known as Kamalasana, and when the legs cross compactly, with either side of the hip moving in strongly toward the midline, it is known as Padmasana.

The reason it is important to practice and get comfortable sitting cross-legged for considerable periods is that this is used in sitting still while keeping the spine erect in the practices of pranayama (breathing techniques) and dhyana (meditation).

Anatomically, to be able to sit cross-legged comfortably requires you to have considerable flexibility in your hamstrings, the back of the hip girdle, and the inner thighs. It also requires you to be able to externally rotate your hip joints. As these areas of the anatomy are large and strong, they can take a long time to stretch and lengthen, allowing you comfort in sitting cross-legged.

It is important to note that the stronger the muscle you're attempting to transform, the more patience you will need. Any excessive effort, either in getting into the pose or in maintaining the pose, can cause serious injury in the hips and legs, especially the knees.

Moreover, the anatomical structure of the hips varies from person to person. This can either make it easier or more difficult for you to sit cross-legged than the next person. So, it is important to not compare your ability to sit cross-legged with others. Be patient and alert as you attempt to sit cross-legged.

Also, if sitting cross-legged is anatomically inaccessible for you, don't think that it is mandatory to your yoga practice. There are several other more accessible seated meditative asanas that, in time, may even help you attain Sukhasana and Padmasana. For example, Vajrasana, or the thunderbolt pose, involves kneeling while keeping your knees together and sitting on your heels. If this is too much of a stretch for your knees, you can place a cushion over your heels to sit more comfortably.

Another alternative to sitting cross-legged is Virasana, or the hero pose. Here you also kneel, keeping your knees together, but instead of sitting on your heels as in Vajrasana, you separate your feet and sit snugly in between your heels. Here, too, if you're unable to sit on the floor between your heels, or if there is even the slightest hint of pain in the knees, you can raise your hips up on blankets, blocks, or bolsters to sit more comfortably in Virasana.

You can also use Gomukhasana, or the cow-faced pose, as a meditative pose or to practice pranayama. This involves sliding one leg under the other and folding both knees so that the ankles rest as close to the outside of the hips as possible. Sitting in Gomukhasana is beneficial in stretching and opening your hips, in relieving chronic knee pain, and in strengthening your ankles and thighs.

Sukhasana, Padmasana, and Gomukhasana are asymmetric poses. So you will need to alternate your legs with either the right or the left leg on top, periodically or in alternate practice sessions. Vajrasana and Virasana are symmetric poses and therefore require no alternation. If you are unable to attain or maintain any of these sitting meditative poses, you can still practice meditation while sitting on a chair. Make sure that the chair is firm, that your spine is straight when seated, and that your feet are flat on the floor or a raised support.

One way to determine if your body is ready for sitting cross-legged is that when you are in the pose, your knees should be at or below your hips. If you find this is not the case, elevate your hips by sitting on blankets or blocks. If elevating your hips destabilizes your knees, you can place additional blankets or bolsters under the knees.

Tension in muscles deep in the abdomen, such as the psoas muscles, is often reflected in tightness in the muscles of the inner thighs called the adductor muscles (adductor brevis, adductor longus, and adductor magnus). When practicing standing poses, it is helpful to imagine releasing the breath down the pelvis and through the legs to relax the muscles of the abdomen and the inner thighs. This can be practiced in all hip opening standing poses such as Virabhadrasana II (warrior pose II), Parshvakonasana (side angle pose), and hip openers such as Padangushtasana I and II (hand to big toe pose) and Supta Baddha Konasana (reclining bound angle pose or cobbler's pose).

Other seated poses that can help you sit cross-legged for longer and with ease and comfort include Janu Sirsasana (head to knee forward fold) and Upavishta Konasana (seated open angle pose).

Practicing a series of forward bends to help you get more comfortable sitting cross-legged must, however, be done judiciously. This is because overemphasizing forward bends can overstretch your lower back. You may prevent overstretching your back after a deep forward bend session by following up with some backbends such as Setu Bandha Sarvangasana (bridge pose), Salabhasana (locust pose), and Bhujangasana (cobra pose).

While you are focused on finding your balance of effort and ease in sitting cross-legged, remember to not tolerate any knee pain. Pain in the knees while crossing your legs can be relieved by placing a rolled towel in the inner crease of the knees before crossing the shins. It is also important to extend your spine while sitting. If this is difficult to achieve in the beginning, try sitting with your back against a wall.

Tight shoulders and a stiff neck can also cause discomfort while sitting cross-legged for long periods. Interlacing your fingers, turning them inside out, and raising your arms overhead, keeping the elbows close to your head (Parvatasana or mountain pose), will help you release any tension in the neck and shoulder.

44. What is the best time and place to practice yoga? Should I practice yoga in front of a mirror?

Although yoga poses strung together in well-thought-out sequences can be practiced at any time of the day, yoga students are generally encouraged to practice at dawn and at dusk for maximal benefit. These timing recommendations are not merely symbolic. At sunrise everything in nature wakes up, and at dusk, everything prepares to sleep. These transition points of the day are accompanied by a change in not only physical energy but also bioenergy. Practicing yoga and meditation at these auspicious times, referred to as Brahma muhurta, literally meaning "the moment of creation," particularly helps in bringing the mind, body, and spirit into quiet focus.

It can be difficult to get up early enough to practice at dawn. This becomes more difficult if you tend to stay up late and have a demanding schedule. Ultimately, you will find your own priorities in life and arrange your schedule accordingly. This may mean aligning your work life around your yoga practice, giving up staying out late with friends, or giving up TV time to get to bed early.

These changes cannot be imposed upon you. You will need to develop your own routines. This is best done organically. This means that you do not "give up" activities you enjoy as you develop your ideal schedule, but you "adopt" activities that you find most beneficial.

Yoga is best practiced on an empty stomach. Therefore, practicing early in the morning before breakfast is a good time. As yoga is a spiritual practice, dedicated practitioners prefer taking a shower before yoga practice. Although taking a shower is optional, emptying your bowels before practice is essential, particularly if you include pranayama in your practice. Pranayama may involve effortful inhalations and exhalations. This can result in undue stress on your internal organs if your bowels are not emptied before practice.

Yoga is best practiced uninterrupted. This means that you should try to dedicate a definite period for your yoga practice alone. Do not schedule your yoga practice in the middle of other activities. For example, taking five minutes from studies or household chores every hour or so during the day to do a yoga asana would be less beneficial than practicing for half an hour at a stretch at a regular time during the day.

Yoga practice needs to be scheduled in such a way that you avoid practicing within two to three hours of a meal. This also makes practicing early in the morning ideal, because you are naturally on an empty stomach in the morning. However, if you must practice in the afternoon or late in the evening, you must make sure to have adequate time between your lunch and afternoon practice or your dinner and your evening practice.

Also, the nature of your practice differs depending on your time of practice. For example, you would not want to practice deep backbends in a late evening practice since this activates your nervous system and increases your metabolism, making it difficult to sleep at night. Although practicing at dawn and dusk is ideal, it is better to use any available time in your schedule for practice than to not practice at all.

The place where you choose to practice yoga should be a clean and quiet place, preferably with fresh air. Some people choose to practice yoga outdoors. Although you can sometimes practice yoga outdoors, particularly if the weather is nice, traditionally, this is not recommended. This is largely because of practical reasons concerning safety. Yoga must be done barefoot and involves lying down on the ground. Therefore, you need to choose a place that is free of insects and germs and physically comfortable. During your entire practice of yoga, unless otherwise directed in cases of specific pranayama techniques, you breathe through the nostrils and not through the mouth. This prevents insects and germs from entering your mouth while you inhale and keeps the in-breath warm, moist, and cleaner than if you were to breathe through your mouth. Moreover, the practice of yoga requires a great deal of concentration and awareness. This is more difficult to attain when you are outdoors.

Moreover, the ground where you practice yoga should be even and not undulating. If you want to practice outside, you will need to find firm plane ground that is not at an incline. Don't practice on bare ground. Use a yoga mat or a blanket on level ground.

Also, if you do decide to practice yoga outdoors, make sure you are not in direct sunlight. Do not practice yoga on a sunlit beach or after sunbathing.

Although some modern schools of yoga conduct classes in heated rooms, this is not normally recommended. Practicing yoga asanas can either generate heat or cool you down. You would therefore want to select a space that is comfortable, preferably where the temperature can be regulated to your comfort levels. Only practice outdoors if you feel safe and comfortable. Do not practice yoga outdoors when the weather is very cold, windy, or hot.

Practicing in front of a mirror is not recommended in yoga except when used as a tool to briefly correct an alignment. Looking into a mirror while practicing yoga draws your mind outward. The aim of yoga is to draw your mind inward. Yoga accomplishes this by sharpening your awareness of where your body and limbs are in space (your proprioceptive sense). Thus, practicing without a mirror is of greater benefit, in the long run, in attaining correct alignment and balance through your internal awareness rather than using the support of cues from a mirror.

However, a mirror is useful in correcting alignment when you suspect your alignment is not quite right. This is best done in the presence of your yoga teacher. You will want to place the mirror such that it is perpendicular to the ground and touching the floor. This way you will be able to see your entire figure in the mirror and correct a misalignment. If the mirror does not touch the floor, you will not be able to see your entire figure in poses such as Sirsasana (headstand). And if the mirror is not perpendicular, you will see your image at a slant, which will not be accurate in gauging your alignment. Once you have corrected your alignment with the aid of the mirror, go back to practicing without it.

45. What equipment do I need at home for my yoga practice and why?

Yoga can be practiced without any equipment at all. The ancient yogis of India who came up with the yoga asanas most likely had no equipment to facilitate their yoga practice.

The point of using equipment in yoga is threefold. The first purpose of using any equipment for yoga practice is to prevent injury. For example, you use a sticky yoga mat so that your feet don't slide, causing you to lose your balance or fall, or you use blankets under your shoulders in Halasana (plow pose) to prevent excess weight and injury in the cervical region at the back of your neck.

The second purpose is to act as therapeutic tools to help you achieve asanas that your body is unable to attain and maintain without help. For example, you use a block under your hands in Trikonasana (triangle pose) when the flexibility in your spine has not yet reached the level of extension where your hands can reach the floor.

And the third purpose is to allow your body to maintain a yoga posture with minimal or no effort on your part with the aim of relaxation and restoration. For example, you use the wall and blankets under your lumbar spine in Viparit Karani (legs up the wall pose) so that you can maintain the pose for a long time with little effort on your part, allowing a passive extension of the upper spine and the muscles of the legs.

Depending on your personal challenges, you might benefit from using props in yoga. These should first be practiced with in class, under the guidance of an able teacher, before you try using them on your own.

The most basic tools for your daily home practice are a sticky mat; four to six blankets a belt, two to four wooden, cork, or foam blocks; bolsters; ace bandages; weights; sandbags; flat boards; and yoga chairs.

A variety of yoga mats, in a range of sizes, designs, materials, and thicknesses, are commercially available in a wide price range. The point of a sticky yoga mat is to prevent your feet from sliding in standing poses and to offer a supportive cushion for seated poses, preventing your body from being too forcefully pushed against a hard floor or sliding on it. Thicker mats offer more support but are also more expensive. Moreover, in some poses, such as Sirsasana (headstand) or supported Dwi pada viparita dandasana (two-legged inverted staff pose), you might be asked to fold your mat. This is not possible if the mat is too thick. You usually store thin yoga mats by rolling them up and leaning them in a corner, although manufacturers of thick yoga mats advise you to keep them laid flat on the ground. Foldable yoga mats are also available and are good to have if you travel a lot. All yoga mats wear out in time as you use them daily, so it is a good idea to replace them before they get too frayed.

The kind of blocks used in alignment-based schools of yoga, such as Iyengar yoga, are made of wood. These are more durable but also more expensive. Cork blocks are less durable but lightweight and cheaper. Foam blocks are the lightest but wear off quicker than the others. Blocks are used creatively in a variety of yoga poses. For example, blocks are used between the soles of the feet in Baddha Konasana (bound angle pose or cobbler's pose) to help open the hips. Blocks are placed under the sacrum in Chatushpadasana (bridge pose) to help you open your chest and raise the pelvis higher.

Bolsters are cylindrical pillows that are plump and round when new but, with time, flatten to an ideal tablet shape. Bolsters are ideally filled with cotton, not polyester. Once bolsters flatten excessively, hardening in the process, they need to be restuffed with fresh cotton. These are creatively used, for example, as a back support in Supta Baddha Konasana (reclining bound angle pose) to extend the spine or in Urdhva Dhanurasana (upward bow pose) as a raised launchpad and comfortable landing platform.

Ace bandages are used as head wraps or eye bags, particularly in restorative asanas and in pranayama to draw the senses inwards. Ace bandages folded and placed over the eyes are light enough to not press down excessively on the eyeballs. The use of eyebags or eye pillows is not recommended in asana or pranayama practice as they are too heavy for the sensitive eyeballs and may cause blurriness of vision afterward.

Cotton belts of various lengths up to seven feet, and widths of half an inch, with square metal clasps are creatively used in a variety of yoga asanas. For example, in Utthita or Supta Padangushtasana I and II (standing or reclining hand to big toe pose I and II), when the hamstrings are not flexible enough for the hands to reach the big toe, the strap is folded and wrapped like the handles of a grocery bag around the feet to achieve balance and equilibrium and to help the hamstrings stretch over time, so that the belt is no longer required.

Folding metal chairs, with crossbars holding both the front legs and the back legs together for sturdiness, are a valuable prop in yoga. These chairs have no back rest and the rim of the back rest is a smooth rounded rim. Yoga chairs are used ingeniously in backbends as well as in standing poses and twists.

You will notice that the goal of using any equipment in yoga is different from that in any other form of exercise, where the primary goal of using an equipment is to increase the effort. For example, you use weights in the gym to increase the effort of muscular contraction.

46. Do I need to lose weight or be more flexible before I can start practicing yoga?

You certainly do not need to lose weight or be more flexible before starting a yoga practice. Yoga is suitable for all body types and all levels of flexibility.

When you go to a yoga class, it is important to not compare yourself to other more advanced practitioners or anyone at all. Yoga is not a competitive sport. Most yoga classes do not have mirrors. This is because yoga aims to develop your own internal sense of how and where your body and limbs are in space (your proprioceptive sense) without the external cue of a mirror. Even when a mirror is used in a yoga class, it is used briefly to show you your alignment and then removed. The absence of mirrors in a yoga class makes it easy to draw the mind inward and not be diverted by other students around you.

It is true that carrying extra weight will make certain poses more challenging for your body. The idea is to push yourself to the edge of your abilities and maintain that edge without going overboard.

Yoga offers tremendous physical and mental strength and resilience, whatever your body weight or level of flexibility. With regular practice your body weight and flexibility with change and adapt to your journey of transformation. Each one of us comes to the yoga mat with some challenge or the other. Yoga helps us work on these challenges with skill, knowledge, and wisdom that has been handed down through the ages. The transformation that occurs through the practice of yoga is subtle and gradual. For example, you may notice making healthier food choices with increased yoga practice because you are calmer and more aware of what foods feel right in your body. Yoga is often described as "skillful action." This involves actions both on and off the mat. As your yoga practice develops, you will notice how the choices you make, both on and off the mat, change your body and mind.

It is also important to avoid the popular yoga myths that social media feeds and sustains. Ignore the images where people twist themselves into crazy pretzels. That is not what yoga is about. Your relationship with yoga must be personal and focused on your own physical and emotional health.

We all must start somewhere. We might not have the ideal weight or suppleness. With practice we improve flexibility, posture, balance, strength, and grace. We also develop fortitude, resilience, and better judgement. You do not need to be able to twist into a pretzel to gain these benefits. Regular practice of the basic poses in yoga lengthens and tones the muscle, strengthens bones, and increases the suppleness of the fascia. A good yoga teacher will help you work through your challenges, whatever they may be, through the creative use of props, ingenious sequences, hands-on assists, and constant encouragement.

The first stage of yoga, known as yamas, includes the practice of santosha, which roughly translates to contentment. In the practice of yoga, it is physically and psychologically important to embrace where you are in the moment. This includes acknowledging the attributes of your current body and mind. The idea is that it is only when we fully inhabit where we are now that we can direct our efforts correctly. However, in the practice of yoga, effort, or tapas, should not be made with an eye on desirable results. Your responsibility, as per the practice of yoga, is to focus on your practice and not on the results. This approach, though counterintuitive to most of Western culture, helps you adhere to your practice without exulting in your achievements or getting demoralized by their lack.

47. How can I get started if I'm too shy or nervous or physically unable to attend a group class?

The great thing about today's world, where we can be on mandatory lock-down in our homes to limit the spread of a pandemic, is that we realize the advantage of technology. So, if you feel shy or nervous about starting yoga with a group of strangers or are physically unable to get to a yoga class, there are several options, including ones where you do not have to leave your home at all.

Online classes: Almost every yoga studio in the country has, in the past couple of months, transitioned into offering online classes. These classes are being offered from beginner levels to advanced levels. As mentioned earlier, there are a number of benefits to in-person classes that are unavailable in online classes, but teachers are finding creative solutions to get around these problems with the help of technology. For example, even though the classes are online and a number of students may be logged on to a class, on their ends, teachers are able to scroll through a gallery of live videos to offer individual feedback.

Friends yoga club: If you are unable to reach a yoga class or are hesitant about attending a yoga class with strangers, you can still take the advantage of a group of friends interested in yoga who might want to take a class with you, offering emotional support. If you have a trusted group of yoga buddies, you might even consider forming an informal yoga club where you practice as a group at each other's homes or at a location convenient for everybody in the group. This form of group learning can be very helpful and fun. You might even consider forming a yoga group in addition to joining a class. Yoga study groups can also be formed online where each member posts a video of their practice and others in the group offer feedback.

Trusted books: Trust yoga references, such as those listed in the bibliography section at the end of this book, can offer a starting point for your yoga practice. Certain yoga books discuss each pose in minute details with step-by-step instructions on how to get into each pose. Although it is difficult to remember all the instructions from a book on a pose and construct a sequence for your practice all on your own, it is possible if you focus on a few poses at a time. These reference books also provide a variety of sequences that you can peruse to find those that are suitable for you.

Expert yoga videos: Instructional videos as well as yoga demonstrations can be purchased and used as source material for practice. In adopting this method, it is important to be extra careful and mindful of your limitations, knowing that you are a beginner whereas the experts demonstrating the poses may have years of practice.

Annual conferences: All major schools of yoga offer national and international annual conferences. These conferences attract thousands of yoga students and experts. If you are unable to attend regular classes, you might opt to attend these annual conferences. You will find a series of classes taught by experts at these conferences together with different discussion panels on various philosophical, didactic, and administrative agendas.

Workshops: Experienced yoga teachers generally travel the world teaching various yoga workshops. Generally, such workshops are open to all levels of students. If you are unable to attend regular yoga classes, you might consider attending one or more yoga workshops a year and work on what you learn at these workshops during your personal practice.

Self-study: Last but not least, self-study is a viable method of learning yoga since the philosophy on which yoga is based proposes that all knowledge lies within and what we learn from external education in classes is nothing but a manifestation of the knowledge that lies within. If you are a beginner, this might not be the best path to take. But if you have a basic knowledge of yoga, it is possible to learn from your own experience and build upon it. This path involves considerable trial and error and may be prone to injuries. Even if you are able to attend classes, your progress will largely depend on your dedicated self-study.

48. How do I improve my posture using yoga?

Activities of our daily lives generally induce us to lean forward, slouch, bend, and jut our heads forward and hunch our shoulders. All yoga asanas bring awareness to the placement of our limbs in space and the alignment of our spine and head. However, the key to improving your posture through yoga is to not limit the awareness and alignment cues to your yoga practice on the mat but carry them on into your daily life.

Contrary to what many people believe, correct posture does not mean having your spine straight as an arrow. Correct posture honors the natural curves of your spine and stacks the weight of your body on the skeletal structures, placing them securely on the weight-bearing part of the soles of your feet under the ankles.

Before you try to correct your posture, however, you need to ascertain the exact problem you have. Your yoga teacher can help you with this. You can also assess your own posture by standing with your back against a wall. When you place the back of your heels close to the wall, your sacrum or tailbone (the upside down triangular bone at the base of your spine), your middle and upper back, and the back of your head should also be in contact with the wall. On the other hand, the lower back and the back of the neck should be a few inches away from the wall, if you have a normal spine. If these spaces at the lower back and neck are more than a few inches away from the wall, your spine is excessively curved. If you must raise your chin to get the back of your head to touch the wall, it means your head juts forward, putting strain on your neck and intervertebral disks.

Posture while standing

Tadasana (mountain pose) is the key to alignment and ease in your posture. Yoga teachers often say that Tadasana is the fundamental pose that allows you to find the correct alignment in all yoga asanas.

Tadasana gives us a number of cues to correct our posture constantly throughout our daily lives, whether we are waiting in the grocery line or standing at the bus stop. Tadasana teaches us to stack our ankles, hips, shoulders, and ears on top of each other without being rigid in our stance. Tadasana keeps us from locking our knees, softening our knees for perfect posture. Tadasana makes us conscious about raising the breastbone, spreading our collarbones sideways, rolling our shoulders out and down our backs, and drawing in the lower tip of the tailbone down and forward to lift your lower abdomen up vertically. Although difficult to grasp in the beginning, Tadasana helps you root your feet firmly into the ground and lengthen your spine vertically upward in a kind of recoiling action.

Posture while sitting

Sitting while engaged in activities like reading or working on the computer makes us unwittingly droop our heads forward and slouch our shoulders forward, causing our postures to sag. When sitting on a chair, we tend to lean our weight on one side. Also, many of us tend to cross our legs when we sit on a chair. This skews the weight distribution at the base of our spines.

The purpose of all the rigorous asanas in yoga is to help you sit comfortably in meditative postures for prolonged periods. Sitting still is not easy. All yoga poses, and particularly the siting poses, teach us how to sit properly, with the least effort and the maximum balance. Depending on the flexibility in your hips, you can practice these sitting asanas: Sukhasana (easy pose), Vajrasana (thunderbolt pose), Virasana (hero's pose), Siddhasana (the accomplished pose), Ardha Padmasana (half lotus pose), Padmasana (lotus pose), Kamalasana (blossoming lotus pose), and Bhadrasana (the gracious pose). In addition to maintaining the spine in its natural curved state, and keeping the chest lifted with the head placed right above the spine, sitting effortlessly for extended periods requires awareness of symmetry. When practicing any of the seated poses or when sitting on a chair, make sure that you are equally balanced on your left and right sitting bones. The strain on the lower back when sitting can be minimized if the thighs slant down toward the knees when you sit. Picture placing a marble at the upper edge of your thigh when you sit. The marble should roll down towards your knees if the angle between your thigh and torso is greater that a right angle. To achieve this, you can elevate your hips on a cushion while sitting in any of the yoga poses or adjust the height of the chair when working at your desk.

Posture while walking

Anecdotal accounts of yoga students show an increased ease of walking with regular practice of yoga. Walking is very beneficial for the body and mind. It oxygenates cells in the body; engages the spine in controlled, rhythmic rotations; and strengthens and tones the quadriceps and hamstrings in the front and back of our thighs. However, postural defects and the need to carry heavy bags on our shoulders and backs cause many of us to tend to walk rigidly, moving solely from the hip sockets and not engaging our core abdominal muscles (psoas muscles). Yoga teaches us the coordination of the movements of the limbs, the spine, and the hip and shoulder girdles to allow grace and ease in our walking postures. For example, in correct walking posture, the shoulders, hips, and knees move from side to side contralaterally. This means that when the right arm moves forward, the left hip moves back and the left knee moves forward. This generates a rhythmic swaying motion and can be practiced on the yoga mat even without moving forward. With increased vigor in movement, the sway of the arms and shoulders increases.

Other postural habits learned on the yoga mat that translate into our walking movement are holding our head right atop the spine without jutting the chin forward or pulling it back; maintaining the natural curves of the spine, turning the tail bone down and hooking it under while lifting the abdomen; and rolling the outer shoulders (deltoid muscles) back and down.

Another interesting way that yoga asanas help improve our walking posture is by translating knowledge gained in one plane of the body into another. For example, if you imagine yourself standing in a doorframe, the plane of the doorframe is the coronal plane of the body. If you now move forward and out of the doorframe, the plane of the direction you are walking in is the sagittal plane of the body. You will notice that an increased awareness of effort and movement in the coronal plane increases your awareness of effort and movement in the sagittal plane. For example, if you do stand in a doorframe and spread your legs such that the outer edges of your feet press into the door frame, and you fold your arms like a goal post in a football field and press your lower arms into the door frame for a few minutes, and then walk forward, you will notice that your awareness of your effort in the coronal plane is translated into an increased awareness of the rhythmic swaying motion in the sagittal plane. This is how the practice of asanas translates our understanding and awareness from one plane of the body to another and from isometric asanas, where muscle tension is increased without shortening the length of the muscle, to dynamic movements such as walking.

The importance of the core in posture

A strong and stable center is important in achieving and maintaining correct posture whether you're sitting, standing, or walking. Although all yoga asanas engage and strengthen the core, some asanas that particularly do so include the following:

1. Boat pose, Navasana
2. Cat pose, Marjariasana
3. Chair pose, Utkatasana
4. Crane pose, Bakasana
5. Scale pose, Tolasana
6. Side plank pose, Vashitasana
7. Four-limbed staff pose, Chaturanga Dandasana
8. Bridge pose, Setu Bandha Sarvangasana
9. Forearm balance, Pincha Mayurasana

Core strength also reduces the likelihood of lower back pain, one of the leading causes of doctor's visits and work and school absences in the world. Good core strength also improves digestion.

Here is a yoga sequence that will focus your attention on the different aspects of your posture:

1. Tadasana (mountain pose)
2. Vrykshasana (tree pose)
3. Marjariasana (cat and cow pose)
4. Uttanasana (standing forward fold)
5. Adho Mukha Shvanasana (downward facing dog pose)
6. Salabhasana (locust pose)
7. Bhujangasana (cobra pose)
8. Dhanurasana (bow pose)
9. Virabhadrasana I (warrior pose I)

49. How can I incorporate mudras into my yoga practice?

You might have noticed you move your hands differently in different states of mind. For example, you may clasp your hands into tight fists when you are angry or rub them together when you're anxious. The gestures of your hands are an expression of your mental state.

"Mudra" is translated as "gesture" or "attitude" in English. The most common forms of mudras are those formed through different configurations of the fingers in one or both hands. For example, the namaskar or namaste mudra is formed by bringing both palms to touch each other such that the circumference of the palms matches exactly. In addition to mudras formed by the hands, mudras can also be formed by the eyes or the entire body.

Mudras are used in hatha yoga to channel or direct energy or to connect two points of energy in the body. For example, energy can be channeled from the base of the spine to the crown of the head. There are five groups of mudra in hatha yoga: hasta mudras (gestures of the hand), mana mudras (gestures of the head), kaya mudras (gestures of the posture), bandhas (gestures that lock energy), and adhara mudras (energetic movements of the pelvic floor).

Hasta mudras can either involve one hand or both hands and are accordingly called ekahasta mudra or dwihasta mudra. The most common dwihasta mudra is the Namaskar mudra, where one folds the palms one on top of each other as in prayer. This is also a form of greeting among Hindus.

Anjali mudra is another hasta mudra where both hands are cupped in the shape of a bowl. This mudra signifies an offering, usually to the divine. Jnana mudra or the gesture of knowledge is formed by each hand with the palms facing upwards, by folding the index finger and curling it to touch the root of the thumb. Jnana mudra is used to induce a contemplative state and is often used in meditative postures.

Sambhavi mudra is a mana mudra that involves the eyes. It is formed by gazing at the eyebrow center. It is used in meditation to induce a state of balance between the right and left side of the body and prepares the mind and body for higher states of consciousness. The mudra is practiced in variations where the eyes are either open or closed. Initially, it is difficult to train the eyes to gaze at the eyebrow center, even with the eyes closed. The eyeballs can only be converged at a certain level of focused concentration. In addition to improving concentration, Sambhavi mudra also strengthens the eye muscles. If practiced incorrectly, Sambhavi mudra causes headache and pain in the eyes. The correct practice involves converging the eyeballs while keeping the gaze and muscles around the eyes relaxed. Therefore, it is encouraged to practice the subtle mudras under the guidance of an experienced teacher who can guide you through the practice in a stepwise and incremental progression of difficulty, thereby preventing injury.

Kaya Mudras are postural mudras that involve asanas, breathing and concentration. Yoga mudra is an example of a Kaya mudra. Yoga mudra is done while sitting in Padmasana (lotus pose) and clasping the wrist of one hand with the other hand behind the back. You then inhale slowly feeling the breath rise from the base of the spine to the middle of the neck. Upon holding the breath in and focusing on the middle of the neck for a few moments, you slowing release the breath while bending forward, coordinating the motion such that the forehead touches the floor when the air is fully expelled from the lungs. Yoga mudra is a preparatory practice for Dhyana or meditation. Physically, it calms the adrenal system, reducing tension and anger while bringing about a sense of tranquility. The Yoga mudra is so called because it unites the internal nature with the external nature.

Bandhas have been discussed in detail in Q32 under pranayamas. Bandhas are a special form of mudra because they are targeted at locking or blocking the outflow of energy from the body. All three bandhas—the Jalandhara Bandha at the neck, the Mooladhara bandha at the base of the pelvic floor and the Uddiyana Bandha that draws the lower abdomen inward and upward—performed together form the Maha Mudra.

Lastly, Adhara mudra directs energy from the pelvic floor upward, toward the brain. Ashwini mudra, literally translated as the gesture of the horse, involves consciously raising the anal sphincter upward in conjunction without straining the surrounding muscles. This is done in conjunction with the breath, namely, while inhaling and retaining the breath inside (Antara Kumbhaka) or while exhaling and retaining the breath outside (Bahiya Kumbhaka). It is considered a preparatory practice for Mooladhara Bandha. Physical benefits of practicing Ashwini Mudra include relief from constipation, piles, and prolapse of the uterus or rectum. To increase the physical and spiritual benefits of Ashwini Mudra, it is often practiced in inverted asanas such as Sarvangasana (shoulder stand).

Scientific studies show that practicing mudras alters neural networks in the brain, both in the short and long term. Mudras offer a path to access our unconscious minds, including our reflexive actions and patterns of habit. The rationale behind the development and practice of mudras has been to create distinct gestures that can give pause to instinctive habits of the body and mind and allow for a more thoughtful and refined consciousness.

❖

Case Studies

1. NICK—FINDING MENTAL AND PHYSICAL BALANCE IN LIFE THROUGH YOGA

Nick is a twenty-two-year-old young man who has recently graduated from college. He has moved to New York from his family home in a small town in the Midwest to explore possibilities in the big city. Nick hopes to find a job in fashion designing. He has been sending out several résumés every day and has been to a few interviews. However, none of the companies he has interviewed with has called him back for a follow-up. He spends long hours applying for jobs, which has been making his lifestyle more and more sedentary. His hamstrings feel tight, and he suffers from frequent headaches due to the uncertainty.

Nick is trying to make new friends in his newly adopted city. He tries to sound hopeful and upbeat when he talks to his family and friends back home. But at times he feels lost and dejected. His dwindling savings and the high cost of living in a big city like New York rattle his sense of financial security. With no responses from prospective employers, he feels rejected and uncertain about his future. He finds his concentration and memory flagging.

Although he has always been a worrier, Nick feels his current levels of anxiety and stress are overwhelming. He grows moody and withdrawn. He finds himself constantly fidgeting and obsessing over minor things. Despite his busy schedule job hunting, he feels disconnected from the world around him and feels he is losing his sense of self and his confidence.

Struggling through his stressful life, Nick is desperately searching for something to balance his stress levels. He feels his life is crumbling around him, and he needs something to hold his body and mind together.

Recently, during a telephone conversation with his friend Marla back home, Nick learns about a thirty-day yoga challenge on YouTube where people practice a yoga sequence and post it online. It comes with the benefit of not costing him anything, unlike his gym membership, and he doesn't need to leave home or buy expensive equipment. He decides to give it a go.

With the requirement of sharing his yoga video with a supportive group of like-minded yoga practitioners as part of the thirty-day yoga challenge, Nick finds a sense of accomplishment and pride, even though he cannot do all the poses perfectly.

Nick watches numerous yoga videos online to learn more about the yoga poses and finds that coordinating his breath with the posture helps him get deeper into the poses with less effort. He soon finds that practicing the short, simple yoga sequences that are assigned to him daily is increasing his flexibility and strength and infusing him with a subtle but definitely positive attitude.

Nick tells his friend Marla during their next phone conversation that he finds that his yoga practice is not only an exercise to power through, but it also connects his body and mind and helps him tap into a sense of self that he had never had access to before.

Nick adds practicing guided yogic meditation or yoga nidra for a few minutes before he goes to bed at night. Nick has always found it difficult to sit still and meditate. His mind would always be flooded with thoughts whenever he tried it. Worse still, when he had tried meditating in the past, he found himself falling asleep if he was too tired or fighting himself in his own head. But practicing scanning his body in the meditative practice of yoga nidra is engrossing and restful because it gives him defined steps that he can do. The sequential steps make it easy to practice yoga nidra regularly. He finds that he no longer needs to fight himself or admonish himself when his mind drifts. He learns that being aware of his drifting mind is part of the process of yogic meditation.

With regular practice and patience, Nick is able to find a sense of balance both on and off his yoga mat. His anxiety and stress levels slowly begin to feel more manageable.

Analysis

Chronic stress and anxiety can wreak havoc on your body. Chemical signals released during chronic stress rewire the brain, sending a person into a downward spiral. Nearly 40 million Americans have been diagnosed with anxiety disorders. Even when clinical symptoms do not manifest, most of us suffer from periodic nervousness and irritability due to the uncertainties and challenges of life. Chronic stress and unchecked anxiety can lead to increased heart rate, hypertension, muscle tension, fatigue, insomnia, panic, and depression. Over long periods, chronic stress and anxiety have been linked to inflammation, migraines, cardiac issues, and even cancer.

Nick, like many young men, found life uncertain and stressful. Additionally, he had a propensity for worrying, which unbalanced his mental health further. Nick's move to a new place increased his physical isolation from all that he had known before. This further increased his anxiety and stress.

Adhering to a simple but regular yoga practice and meditation session helped Nick find his mental balance and gave him an optimistic outlook on life. Here is the simple yoga sequence Nick practiced at the very beginning that helped calm his anxiety and find his center during turmoil:

1. Supine head-to-big-toe pose (Padangushtasana)
2. Supine twist (Jathara Parivartanasana)
3. Cat pose (Marjariasana)
4. Balancing table pose (Dandayaman Bhramanasana)
5. Plank pose (Phalankasana)
6. Downward dog pose (Adho Mukha Shvanasana)
7. Warrior II (Virabhadrasansa II)
8. Triangle pose (Trikonasana)
9. Tree pose (Vrykshasana)
10. Bound angle pose (Baddha Konasana)
11. Camel pose (Ushtrasana)
12. Bow pose (Dhanurasana)
13. Supported shoulder stand (Salamba Sarvangasana)
14. Corpse pose (Shavasana)

2. CARL—TRANSITIONING BETWEEN ATHLETICS AND YOGA

Carl is a twenty-six-year-old athlete. He has always been hardworking, a truly type-A personality, task-driven and adrenaline addicted. Earlier he had trained as a weightlifter, but a skiing injury severed the ACL ligament in his knee. After a long, difficult recovery, Carl was a regular at the gym and had taken up a rigorous CrossFit training regimen. However, as Carl regained his strength, he found himself becoming very tight and inflexible.

At the suggestion of a friend, Carl decided to join a yoga class at the gym. Carl had expected the yoga class to be easy and relaxing, but he was surprised to find that seemingly easy-looking poses such as downward facing dog pose, which almost everyone in the class can do without breaking into a sweat, were next to impossible for him. Being the trained athlete that he was, Carl put in more effort to will his body into the yoga postures. He practiced both in the morning before going to the gym and in the evening at home before dinner.

Within a few weeks, Carl developed intense pain in his knees, hamstrings, and shoulder joints and got increasingly frustrated with his progress in yoga. It appeared to him that the more effort he put into his practice, the less progress he was making. In fact, he was injuring himself in ways he'd never done before in his years of training as a weightlifter and skier.

Discussing his experience with yoga with another friend who was also a weightlifter, he found his friend had been injured in yoga class at his gym as well. His friend told him he thought yoga could do more harm than good when practiced incorrectly. Taking his friend's advice, he accompanied his friend to an alignment-based therapeutic yoga class across town.

He told his yoga teacher about his shoulder injury and how he had found it difficult to do simple poses at the yoga class at the gym that primarily was a flow-type yoga class.

The therapeutic yoga teacher talked to Carl about the approach they are going to adopt for his session. The teacher told Carl, although it may be difficult for him, he has to take a step back from his effortful competitive attitude. "Often the thing you need most is what you want to do the least," said the yoga teacher.

Carl noticed that the therapeutic yoga teacher focused on his shoulder mobility rather than his shoulder strength. His teacher told him that the shoulder joint is the most mobile joint in the body. Therefore, for nonathletes, he usually begins with poses that strengthen the shoulder joint. However, athletic training already provides strength to the crucial shoulder muscles developing the trapezius and deltoid muscles disproportionately. Excessive overhead lifting also reduces the mobility of the shoulder joint and increases rounding in the upper back.

As Carl was unable to bend his elbow and clasp his palms behind his back as is done in Gomukhasana (cow face pose), a classical pose used to increase shoulder mobility, the teacher attempted to increase his shoulder mobility using a preparatory movement.

The teacher asked Carl to sit cross-legged on a couple of blankets and hold a yoga belt with both hands such that the hands are almost as wide as his knees. Keeping his elbows as straight as possible he was to raise his arms above his head as he inhaled and, with an exhalation, bring the arms way down behind his back, keeping the strap taut and without moving his hands on the strap. Carl found that as he made the bend with his arms above his head and down his back, there came a point where he felt he could not rotate his arms anymore. He was stuck. His teacher asked him to relax his effort in getting through this point. "Rather than forcing your way through, see whether you can breathe into it," said the teacher. Initially, Carl could not rotate his arms beyond a certain point, but as he continued to attend the therapeutic yoga class week after week, he saw that it was possible to release his instinctive muscular effort. With time the mobility in his shoulder joints increased, and this allowed him to not only rotate his arms over his head and behind his back but also made it possible for him to clasp his palms on his spine in Gomukhasana.

Carl also noticed that working with his yoga therapist was very different from the yoga flow class he attended at his gym. Whereas at the gym, the teacher moved in quick succession from one pose to the other, and everyone else followed along, the yoga therapist emphasized holding a pose for extended periods and adjusting the pose to find the perfect alignment. This gave Carl the time and opportunity to understand his body and his range of motion, both in terms of the advantages of his years of weightlifting and his restricted flexibility. This helped him not only approach his yoga practice with greater patience and humility but also improve his performance at the gym.

Unlike the flow yoga teacher at the gym, who taught primarily by demonstration and broad verbal cues, the yoga therapist gave Carl subtle cues that compelled him to think and continuously adjust his physical alignment and mental attitude. Carl found himself paying close attention to his feet when he did the standing poses. He noticed that when he turned his feet outward, his lower back felt tight and restricted, and when he turned them inward, his lower back felt broad and spacious. But it was not possible to stand pigeon-toed, either in yoga or off the mat. So, he challenged himself to keep his upper thighs turned inward while his feet were parallel, so that his lower back still found the broadness it had with his toes turned inward. In time, Carl found this not only gave him greater balance in the standing poses but also improved his posture.

Analysis

Training in specific athletic sports develops certain muscles disproportionately to the rest of the body. This excessive localized muscular strength restricts mobility because mobility requires the coordinated action of diverse muscle groups. Therefore, it is often quite difficult for an athlete to practice yoga, particularly in flow-type classes that offer limited alignment cues and assume a certain level of flexibility from the students. Athletes thrown into high-powered Vinyasa yoga classes often end up injuring themselves or abandoning yoga altogether. This is unfortunate. Athletes seeking to practice yoga would benefit from working with a yoga therapist or an alignment-based yoga class that focuses more on mobility than strength building. Moreover, athletes often come to yoga classes with prior injuries and internal scar tissues. A slow, alignment-based approach that takes into consideration the advantages and disadvantages of the athlete's body allows athletes to recover from past injuries and find greater balance and harmony.

Here is a yoga sequence that Carl practiced slowly with a focus on alignment that improved his shoulder mobility as well as the pain in his lower back and neck:

1. Supported Shavasana with his calves raised on the seat of a chair, arms extended and weighed down with sandbags (corpse pose)
2. Supta Padangushtasana I (hand to big toe pose I)
3. Supta Padangushtasana II (hand to big toe pose II)
4. Adho Mukha Shvanasana (downward-facing dog pose)
5. Uttanasana (standing forward bend)
6. Bharadvajasana (Sage Bharadvaja's twist)
7. Gomukhasana (cow face pose)
8. Trikonasana (triangle pose)
9. Utthita Parsvakonasana (extended side angle pose)
10. Ardha Chandrasana (half-moon pose)
11. Paschima Namaskarasana (greeting the west pose)
12. Virasana (hero's pose)

3. NADIA—EASING MENSTRUAL CRAMPS USING YOGA

Nadia's friend Asha called to confirm their tennis class at the local recreation center that evening. But Nadia told her friend she couldn't make it to class that week. Nadia is seventeen and has been dreading the time of her monthly periods since they started when she was twelve. Although mostly regular, Nadia's periods start with a light flow that lasts for about three days and then stops, only to start again with a heavy flow that can last anywhere from four to seven days. Nadia's periods are accompanied by debilitating abdominal cramps, diarrhea, stiffness, and headaches.

Nadia usually stays home from school during her period because of the pain and fatigue. Also, Nadia finds her periods are often accompanied by either diarrhea or constipation. She detests leaving home during her periods. However, she is in high school now, and taking days off isn't as easy as it had been earlier. Once, when Nadia returned to school after an absence of over a week due to a particularly rough cycle, her teacher referred her to the school counselor.

Nadia went to see the school counselor, who advised her to talk to her gynecologist about her problems with her period. Nadia's gynecologist advised her to take analgesics at the start of her menstrual bleeding and informed her of other preventative measures such as avoiding caffeine and alcohol as well as using a heating pad for her lower back or abdomen and resting when needed. As Nadia's gynecologist was also well informed about the complementary medicine and the beneficial effects of therapeutic yoga for the management of menstrual problems, she also gave Nadia a flyer for an alignment-based yoga class.

The gynecologist also told Nadia that although there is a lack of good medical studies on the effects of yoga in managing menstrual issues, based on her medical experience, she knew of substantial anecdotal evidence when a regular practice of yoga has brought relief to patients who had been suffering chronic problems such as prolonged bleeding and pain in the lower abdomen, thighs, back, neck, and shoulders.

Nadia decided to try yoga. She had not attended a yoga class before and was hesitant to talk about her problems in a class. So, Nadia sought out a private yoga instructor who would give her yoga lessons at her own apartment once a week.

During her first session with the yoga instructor, Nadia told her teacher about her issues and reasons for turning to yoga. Her teacher, in turn, asked her several questions about her age, lifestyle, level of suppleness and strength, posture and manner of walking, injuries and surgeries, and whether she has had any prior practice of yoga. After a detailed discussion, her teacher advised her on getting some yoga props such as six to ten blankets, a couple of bolsters, four yoga blocks, and a strap or belt, in addition to the mat that Nadia had already acquired.

For the first few weeks, Nadia worked with her instructor to start some standing poses to build strength and gain some confidence in yoga itself. Nadia's teacher modified the classical asanas with the use of props so that the poses became more accessible for her current level of strength and suppleness. Using the props also helped Nadia understand the alignment required in specific asanas and helped her find balance. Gradually, Nadia found her body relaxing into the poses rather than attempting to attain the poses through a lot of muscular effort. With continued practice, she found an increase in the range of motion and the strength in her muscles and joints, which allowed her to hold restorative poses for prolonged periods.

Slowly, Nadia's teacher introduced her to sequences designed specifically to address her issues of painful menstrual cramps. When Nadia was able to regularly practice these sequences, she saw a reduction in the pain and cramps that accompanied her monthly period. In time, Nadia also noticed a reduction in the duration of her periods.

Analysis

Dysmenorrhea is a common problem among women worldwide. Consumption of analgesics and rest is the normal strategy for coping in such circumstances. However, scientific studies show the efficacy of yoga in dealing with the range of symptoms accompanying dysmenorrhea. Studies report significant improvement in pain symptoms, gastrointestinal symptoms, cardiovascular symptoms, and urogenital symptoms in controlled studies where patients have undergone an intervention program consisting of yoga asanas and meditation.

Menstruation is accompanied by the release of prostaglandins, which are hormone-like substances that help to contract the uterine wall. Practicing Supta Baddha Konasana (reclining bound angle pose) regularly, and particularly during your period, soothes the digestive system and provides relief from painful menstrual cramps.

Asanas that involve twists are also recommended during menstruation. Twists such as Supta Bharadvajasana (reclining pose of sage Bharadvaj) stretch the lower back and hips while infusing the digestive system with fresh blood flow.

Effortful inversions are usually not recommended during your period, however relaxing inversions such as Viparit karani (legs up the wall pose) or Setu bandha sarvangasana (supported bridge pose) help promote focus and clarity while improving circulation and digestion and lowering blood pressure. Supported inversions also have a calming effect on the nervous system, reducing anxiety and depression.

This yoga sequence relieves menstrual cramping and discomfort:

1. Baddha konasana (bound angle pose)
2. Adho Mukha Virasana (child's pose)
3. Janu sirsasana (head of the knee pose)

4. Upavishta konasana (seated wide angled pose)
5. Paschomottanasana (intense stretch of the west pose)
6. Supported Uttanasana (standing forward fold)
7. Setu bandha sarvangasana (supported bridge pose)
8. Supta baddha konasana (reclined bound angle pose)
9. Viparita Karani (legs up the wall pose)

4. HANNAH—A COMFORTABLE PREGNANCY AND SMOOTH DELIVERY WITH PRENATAL YOGA

Hannah is a twenty-three-year-old young woman pregnant with her first child. She has a family history of hypertension and diabetes but is in good health.

Hannah has been going to yoga classes once or twice a month ever since she left high school. She does not practice yoga regularly but has always led a fairly active lifestyle. For the past couple of years, she has been working at a medical billings department, which involves working at a desk for over eight hours a day. This has caused her to gain some weight, but she has been trying to shed the weight by trying out different diet regimens, hiking, cycling, and working out at the gym during the weekends. When she is able to stick to her diet, she loses a few pounds but soon gains them back again.

Hannah's marriage a couple of years ago to her high school sweetheart, Bob, soon after she had started her job at the medical billings department, has increased her responsibilities; and finding time for herself, whether to exercise or simply to take it easy, has become increasingly difficult.

Last week Hannah learned of her pregnancy, which has filled her life with hope and joy. It has also made her think about changes she needs to make to her lifestyle to retain her strength and flexibility through her pregnancy and prepare for a smooth delivery.

Her past interests in hiking and cycling did not seem feasible to her during her pregnancy, so she consulted her gynecologist for advice. Familiar with her medical history, her gynecologist recommended she attend prenatal yoga classes.

While researching online, Hannah found a yoga studio only a block away from her home that offered prenatal yoga classes. Hannah was only a month and a half into her pregnancy and had not even started showing yet. So, she wondered whether it was the right time for her to attend the prenatal yoga class. She called the yoga studio and talked to a senior teacher, who told her that she can start attending yoga classes as early in her pregnancy as she likes. However, she said, if she is not feeling well and is going through morning sickness, which is common in the first trimester, she should wait until she is past this phase.

Hannah began attending the prenatal yoga class at the local studio and noticed that although her pregnancy was not noticeable on the outside, she already felt different on the inside. She took the advice of her yoga teacher and paid close attention to how her body felt while practicing the poses. As her pregnancy progressed, she learned to tune in and respect the cues her body gave her. She also noticed that keeping to a regular yoga practice reduced her stress levels and increased her comfort.

On days that she did not feel like attending a yoga class at the studio, Hannah practiced at home. To help her with her home practice, Hannah asked her teacher for yoga sequences and modifications of yoga poses that she could do at home. She bought some props, including additional blankets and bolsters that helped her practice the modified poses at home. Her teacher also advised her to listen carefully to what her body wants on a particular day and not try to advance her yoga practice at this time by overstretching or twisting in yoga poses.

Hannah initially focused on hip-opening poses in her daily yoga practice. These poses create flexibility in the hip that can make giving birth easier. Hip-opening poses that Hannah's teacher recommended she practice regularly included Eka Pada Rajakapotasana (pigeon pose), Virabhadrasana II (warrior pose II), Trikonasana (triangle pose), Ardha Chandrasana (half-moon pose), Baddha Konasana (bound angle pose), and Agnistambhasana (firelog pose).

The hip-opening poses gave Hannah a great deal of relief as her pregnancy advanced, and she was able to manage occasional lower back discomfort and stiffness. These poses not only stretched her thighs and groin but also her lower back relieving pain.

Hannah also practiced some poses that involved stretching sideways. These included Parighasana (gate pose) and supported Vashishthasana (supported side plank pose). These side stretches gave Hannah relief in the abdominal area, which was starting to feel crowded as the pregnancy advanced.

To keep her strength up, Hannah practiced a modified version of the sun salutation well into her third trimester. She widened her stance in standing poses to make room for her growing baby bump, particularly in poses that involved bending forward.

Later in pregnancy, when Hannah was told that her baby was not in an optimal position for birth, with its head down and its back to her belly, her prenatal care provider, a yoga student herself, asked her to practice Chakravakasana (cat-cow pose) while she manually assisted her in turning the breech baby.

In addition to advising Hannah on poses she should practice during her pregnancy, her yoga teacher also advised her on poses and movements she should avoid, such as overstretching, twisting her torso, jumping into poses, fast breathing, inversions, back-bending, abdominal-strengthening poses that contract the abdominal region, poses that involve lying on the belly or back, and yoga styles that are vigorous or involve raising your body's core temperature.

Despite a family history of hypertension and diabetes, Hannah was able to maintain normal blood pressure and blood glucose levels through-out her pregnancy. Her delivery went smoothly, and she gave birth to a healthy baby boy.

Analysis

Pregnancy is a period of high stress accompanied by unique physical and psychological demands. Maternal stress conditions the environment in the womb and has negative effects on the growing fetus as well. These effects may be retained throughout the growing years of the child and into adulthood. For example, maternal stress during pregnancy has been linked to slow maturation; abnormal behavioral responses; reduced learn-ing, memory, and attention; and decrease in brain volume.

Yoga provides a way to manage maternal discomfort, stress, and pain during pregnancy and birth, promoting quality of life and optimizing infant health and development. Physical exercises were once discouraged during pregnancy. However, recent studies show that the practice of prenatal yoga during pregnancy is not only safe but also helps boost self-confidence, flexibility, strength, and coping strategies in expectant mothers.

As women have specific needs and limitations during pregnancy, an individually customized yoga sequence incorporating the practices of asanas (physical postures), pranayama (breathing techniques), and dhyana (meditation) shows the best results. Certain movements and poses are to be avoided during pregnancy. For example, the hormone relaxin, secreted by the body during pregnancy, makes pregnant women vulnerable to over-stretching. Therefore, it is important to not push your limit in yoga poses during pregnancy, as this may cause pulled ligaments or tendons, which take a long time to heal. Similarly, twisting poses can compress internal organs, including the uterus, and so should be avoided. Jumping into poses is obviously discouraged because it can jolt the fetus in the womb. Even during early pregnancy, jumping into poses is to be avoided because it poses a risk of dislodging the fertilized egg from the uterine wall.

Instead of practicing breath retentions or rapid inhalations and exhala-tions (e.g., in Kapalabhati or breath of fire), deep inhalations through the nose and long exhalations through the mouth are recommended instead during pregnancy. This breathing form is also applied during the birthing process. Learning to focus on the breath is a valuable tool that can help keep you grounded in the present and manage labor pains. Although inversions don't put the fetus at risk, it is recommended to avoid them to prevent falling. However, supported and modified inversions can be helpful in preventing or reducing the likelihood of premature birth. Poses that involve lying on the belly or the back are to be avoided to prevent discomfort. Shavasana or corpse pose can be modified by lying on the side using blankets or bolsters to make yourself comfortable. Importantly, practices such as Bikram yoga that involve raising your core body temperature are not recommended during pregnancy.

5. JINZHE—DEALING WITH TRAUMA THROUGH YOGA

Jinzhe is currently a twenty-five-year-old intensive care unit nurse at Walter Reed hospital in Washington, DC. He had enlisted in the military at age eighteen and was deployed to Afghanistan in combat service three times before he left the army at twenty-three. He now works rotating shifts at the hospital and leads a highly regular life. He is married to his beautiful wife, Sasha, and they are expecting their first child early next year.

Although on the surface Jinzhe appears calm and settled in his lifestyle, certain triggers can still bring back terrible memories of the time he was in the military. He is also plagued by nightmares that rarely allow him restful sleep. His lack of sleep and rotating shifts at the hospital also cause Jinzhe to eat in a haphazard manner, leading to weight gain. Even though he eats regularly, he has been having trouble digesting his food and has developed some food allergies. He feels constantly on edge.

Last summer, when their whole family including both his and Sasha's parents went to the National Mall to enjoy the Fourth of July fireworks, Jinzhe found himself gasping for air by the end of the show. Although he managed to keep a superficially calm persona until late at night, once he was in bed, the terrors, flashbacks, and nightmares returned. Sasha drove him to the emergency room, where he was given Zoloft to calm him down.

When Jinzhe experiences one of his episodes, he feels as though the light changes and he is not even in the room. Triggers are hard to identify and avoid. Jinzhe rarely watches the news or reads the daily paper. Before he was deployed, Jinzhe had prided himself on staying abreast of current affairs. But now news from anywhere around the world that is ravaged by war reminds him of his own experiences. He can never be sure what will trigger an episode, though. Sometimes it can be as simple as a car backfiring or a surprise pat on the back from a friend. He had expected to enjoy the fireworks display at the mall, and yet it triggered a chain reaction in his mind and body that he could not control.

Jinzhe has been scouring the internet for a practice for fitness and relaxation that can be done anywhere and anytime. He hopes that in addition to therapy, a regular fitness practice will help him regain his optimal weight and help him sleep easily.

Last winter Jinzhe volunteered to be part of a research trial at the Walter Reed Army Medical Center that aimed to investigate the role of yoga's therapeutic potential on sleep and depression in PTSD patients. As part of the trial, Jinzhe learnt the technique of yoga nidra, also called yogic sleep. After the trial, when Jinzhe was asked to describe the effect of the intervention on his day-to-day life, he simply told the reporter that the program has helped him identify little chunks of his life that he can work on. Clinical parameters that were measured before and after the six-week yoga therapy program showed an increase in Jinzhe's immune cell counts and a decrease in the plasma levels of the stress hormone cortisol.

Jinzhe found that yoga helped him re-establish a sense of control over his body and his time. Regular practice of breathing techniques such as Sudarshan Kriya allowed him to use these tools when he sensed a flashback or a panic attack coming. The practice of yoga nidra increased his endurance of situations beyond his control. Jinzhe also saw the benefit of repeating a simple phrase, or a mantra, either audibly or silently in his mind as he went about his daily work.

It has been five years now since his last deployment. He has been practicing yoga and meditation for the past four years. Jinzhe still recalls his rigorous military training and his horrifying experience in Afghanistan. But he now realizes that the aggressive response to threat and the inherent anger that was instilled in him as a result of his military experience are things he can let go. He has sleeping better lately and hopes to stop taking antidepressants soon.

Analysis

Yoga is popularly practiced for reducing stress levels and to promote a sense of calm. It is especially beneficial for veterans suffering from post-traumatic stress disorder (PTSD). PTSD is a chronic malaise that drains an individual's fortitude and energy to cope with life. As per recent estimates, nearly 8 percent of all adults in the United States are battling

PTSD. A large percentage of veterans suffer from PTSD, even if they do not fight at the frontlines. Leaving their families at a fairly young age to support various military missions around the world, working on airplanes, processing documentation regarding the deaths of fellow soldiers, as well as active combat all take a toll on young soldiers.

The *Diagnostic and Statistical Manual of Mental Disorders* categorizes PTSD as a trauma- and stressor-related disorder caused by the exposure of an individual to a traumatic of stressful event. Individuals suffering from PTSD are unable to put the memory of the traumatic event behind them. Instead, they continue to re-experience the trauma through vivid memories, nightmares, flashbacks, emotional distress, and physical reactivity. Individuals suffering from PTSD tend to avoid things that they associate with the trauma and may be unable to recall details of the traumatic event. PTSD is also associated with negative thoughts, self-blame, decreased interest in activities, feelings of isolation, irritability, aggression, hypervigilance, increased startle reaction, and difficulty in concentrating and sleeping.

A meta-analysis of nearly twenty randomized control trials including over 1,600 participants showed that meditation and yoga are promising complementary approaches in the treatment of PTSD among adults. The yoga studies included in the meta-analysis examined trauma-informed yoga programs and included Kripalu-based yoga, Kundalini yoga, and deep stretching and breathing exercises. Trauma-informed Kripalu and Kundalini yoga are based on hatha yoga principles that emphasize the use of asanas, awareness of breathing, and the connection between the body and mind.

In addition to the profound effect that prolonged practice of yoga has on the body and mind, there are several fringe advantages of adopting yoga in the treatment of PTSD. For instance, complementary health approaches such as yoga are usually offered in a group format that encourage participants to take an active role. Certified instructors dedicated to serving communities in need, such as veterans, are widely available given the popularity of yoga in recent decades in the United States. As there is no need for highly specialized equipment, participants can practice the yoga and meditation techniques both at home and at regular classes, thereby yielding faster results in relieving symptoms of PTSD. Moreover, participants are encouraged to use the breathing and alignment principles that they learn and discover in their own practice "off the mat" and incorporate these practices in all aspects of their lives. This increases the frequency of their use and the intensity of their effect.

Other studies of female patients show regular hatha yoga practice reduces the frequency of intrusive, negative thoughts, the intensity of jangled nerves as well as improve heart-rate variability. Heart-rate variability is a marker for a person's ability to calm herself.

Here is a simple body scanning technique that Jinzhe practices as part of his yoga nidra routine:

1. Lie down on your yoga mat or on a blanket, in Shavasana.
2. Feel the weight of your body completely supported by the earth.
3. Repeat a phrase that you find soothing and calming, such as "I am filled with love and peace."
4. Gently but quickly guide your awareness through your body, relaxing the skin and muscles of each area as you move through the entire body. Follow a certain logical pattern in the movement of awareness through your body. For example, move from the soles of your feet to your toes, to your ankles, calves, knees, thighs, and so on until you reach the top of your head.
5. Once you have scanned your entire body a few times, bring your attention to your breath.
6. Slowly externalize the mind, becoming aware of surroundings once again.
7. Gently turn to one side, sit up, and open your eyes.

Glossary

Abhyasa (Sanskrit): dedicated practice.

Adho- (Sanskrit): a prefix that indicates downward.

Agni (Sanskrit): fire.

Ahimsa (Sanskrit): nonviolence.

Anjali (Sanskrit): a dwihasta mudra or two-handed gesture cupping both hands in the shape of a bowl that indicates an offering.

Anusara (Sanskrit): following your heart, or flowing with nature; also a particular school of Hatha yoga.

Asana (Sanskrit): literally translates as "seat" but currently used to mean physical postures or poses.

Asana (Sanskrit): literally meaning "to be seated comfortably," it is the third limb of the eight-limbed path of yoga.

Ashtanga (Sanskrit): literally translates as "eight (ashta)-limbed (anga)"; refers to the eightfold path of yoga.

Atman (Sanskrit): the true, eternal self, commonly translated as "spirit" or "soul."

Autonomic nervous system: the part of the peripheral nervous system that innervates the internal organs such as the liver, kidney, blood vessels, and so on and works without an individual's conscious effort.

Ayama (Sanskrit): to stretch or extend.

Baddha (Sanskrit): bound.

Baka (Sanskrit): crane.

Bandha (Sanskrit): internal muscular locks that, when engaged, support toning and lifting of areas of the body.

Bhagavad Gita: a 700-verse subsection (chapters 23–40) of the 100,000-verse Indian Hindu epic Mahabharata, written by Vyasa in the fourth century.

Bhakti (Sanskrit): literally translated as "devotion," it is also a path in yoga that is based on love for the divine.

Bhastrika (Sanskrit): popularly known as the "bellowing breath" technique, it is a pranayama where the abdomen is made to thrust in and out like a bellow with every exhalation and inhalation through the nostrils.

Bhramar (Sanskrit): bee.

Bhuja (Sanskrit): arms.

Bikram yoga: also called hot yoga, it is a sequence of twenty-six vigorous poses done in a heated room.

Brahman (Sanskrit): used in the nominative, singular, neutral gender, it refers to the concept of ultimate reality and is central to Hindu and Vendanta philosophy.

Chakra (Sanskrit): literally translated as "circles," chakras indicate energetic focal points along the spine. There are seven chakras along the length of the spine: the root chakra (Muladhara), the sacral chakra (Svadhishthan), the naval chakra (Manipura), the heart chakra (Anahata), the throat chakra (Vishuddi), the third eye chakra (Ajna), and the crown chakra (Sahasrara).

Core: anatomically, the midsection or torso of the body that functions as a stabilizer and includes the belly or abdomen, hips, and the mid and lower back.

Danda (Sanskrit): staff or stick.

Diaphragm: a dome-shaped muscle that separates the chest cavity from the abdomen in mammals, its contraction causes it to well downward, causing the space in the chest cavity to increase while its relaxation causes it to rise upward, reducing the space in the chest cavity and enabling breathing.

Drishti (Sanskrit): literally meaning "sight," it refers to the gazing technique practiced while holding a yoga pose.

Flight-or-fight response: first described by Walter Bradford Cannon, this is a physiological acute stress reaction that occurs when a person encounters an event that is either physically or mentally terrifying.

Guru (Sanskrit): a word that means "teacher" but can also mean heavy, grave, or serious.

Hasta (Sanskrit): hands.

Hatha yoga (Sanskrit): one meaning is "willful" or "effortful" and indicates yoga where effort is needed; another meaning is based on the combination of "Ha," meaning the sun and "tha" meaning the moon indicating balance and equilibrium.

Hatha Yoga Pradipika (Sanskrit): a text compiling yoga asana, pranayamas, kriyas and bandhas, written by Svatmarama in the fifteenth century.

Intercostal muscles: groups of muscles found between the ribs that help move the ribs in a bucket-handle motion (i.e., upward and outward) with every inhalation.

Jivamukta (Sanskrit): a combined word derived from the root words "jiv," meaning "to breathe" or "to live," and "mukta," meaning "liberated," jivamukta means an individual who is "liberated while still living."

Jivatma (Sanskrit): derived from the root word "jiv," meaning "to breathe" or "to live," jivatma refers to a living being.

Kapalabhati (Sanskrit): a pranayama, popularly known as the "breath of fire," that literally means "head perception"; kapala = head or skull and bhati = perception or knowledge.

Karma (Sanskrit): literally translated as "action," it is also a path in yoga based on focus on one's work without seeking results.

Kona (Sanskrit): angle.

Kumbhaka (Sanskrit): literally meaning "vessel," kumbhaka refers to the retention of the breath either inside the body after an inhalation (anatara kumbhaka) or outside the body after exhalation (bahiya kumbhaka).

Kundalini (Sanskrit): literally meaning "coiled," kundalini refers to the latent feminine energy that is believed to lie "coiled" at the base of our spines at the Muladhara chakra. Kundalini yoga is a method of asana (postures) and dhyana (meditation) directed toward the rise and release of the kundalini energy at the base of our spines.

LDL or low-density lipoproteins: sometimes called bad cholesterol because their increase leads to a buildup of cholesterol and plaques in arteries as opposed to HDL, high-density lipoproteins, dubbed good cholesterol.

Manana (Sanskrit): reflecting, considering, weighing, assimilating.

Mantra (Sanskrit): a sound, word or phrase that is repeated to promote concentration in meditation.

Meta-analysis: the statistical procedure for combining data from multiple studies.

Moksha (Sanskrit): release or liberation.

Mudra (Sanskrit): a gesture, mostly commonly of the hands, but also of the head or the entire body that is associated with a particular state of the mind.

Nada yoga (Sanskrit): a form of yoga based on the practice of regulating of sound vibrations.

Nadi (Sanskrit): literally translated as "channel," "stream," or "flow," nadis specifically signify the flow of the life force or prana through the body. According to yoga texts, there are 350,000 nadis that course to the different layers of the human body. The three most commonly known nadis are Ida, Pingala, and Sushumna that run on either side and through the spinal cord.

Namaste/Namaskar (Sanskrit): a respectful greeting said with joined palms in front of the chest when you meet someone. It literally means, "I bow to the divine in you."

Niddhyasana (Sanskrit): realizing the truth of a matter.

Niyama (Sanskrit): universal duties or observances described in the Yoga Sutras as Saucha (cleanliness), Santosha (contentment), Tapas (discipline), Svadhyaya (self-study), and Ishvara Pranidhana (surrendering to a higher power).

Om (Sanskrit): also written as "aum," it is a spiritual sound in Hinduism that symbolizes the ultimate reality or the sum total of all that exists. When chanted Om vibrates at a frequency of 432 Hz, which is identical to the vibrational frequency in all natural things.

Pada (Sanskrit): foot.

Parasympathetic nervous system: a part of the peripheral autonomic nervous system that is responsible for inhibiting body processes, such as heart rate, blood pressure, breathing, and so on.

Parivritta (Sanskrit): revolved.

Parshva (Sanskrit): sideways.

Paschima (Sanskrit): west.

Patanjali (Sanskrit): Patanjali was an Indian sage who lived around 150 BCE and is believed to be the author of a number of important Sanskrit works on yoga, medicine, and grammar. Patanjali is believed to have written the Yoga Sutras.

Prana (Sanskrit): in Hindu philosophy, including yoga, Indian medicine, and martial arts, prana is described as the life force that emanates from the cosmos and connects all elements.

Pranava (Sanskrit): the name for the Sanskrit symbol of Om (ॐ), literally meaning "to sound loudly."

Pranayama (Sanskrit): derived from the words "prana," meaning "life force," and "yama," meaning "control," pranayama is a type of meditation that involves the regulation of the breath. It is also the fourth limb of the eight-limbed path of yoga.

Purva (Sanskrit): east.

Raja (Sanskrit): literally translated as "royal," it is also a path in yoga that focuses on meditation and skill in action.

Randomized control trials: scientific experiments that aim to reduce bias by randomly allocating subjects to different test and control or placebo groups, treating them differently, and then comparing their quantitative response.

Sacrum: a large, wedge-shaped vertebra at the bottom of the spine that supports the weight of the upper body.

Saraswati (Sanskrit): Hindu goddess of knowledge.

Shakti (Sanskrit): feminine power.

Shanti (Sanskrit): peace, rest, calmness, tranquility, or bliss.

Shastra (Sanskrit): spiritual texts.

Shravana (Sanskrit): active listening.

Shvana (Sanskrit): dog.

Siddhi (Sanskrit): perfection, accomplishment, attainment, or success.

Sruti (Sanskrit): literally meaning "what is heard," this describes sacred spiritual works that were transmitted by ancient sages to their disciples through chanting and recitation or word of mouth and were later written down. Works of "sruti" are in contrast to works of "smriti" or that which is remembered and then written.

Sudarshan Kriya (Sanskrit): literally meaning "proper vision through purifying action," Sudarshan Kriya is an advanced form of rhythmic, periodic breathing that is performed at a progressively increasing pace.

Sukhino bhava (Sanskrit): a form of greeting or blessing meaning "may you be happy."

Svadhyaya (Sanskrit): self-study, i.e., study of one's own inherent tendencies, habits, affinities etc. as well as studying spiritual texts with the aim of understanding oneself better.

Sympathetic nervous system: a part of the peripheral autonomic nervous system that is responsible for stimulating body processes, such as heart rate, blood pressure, breathing, and so on.

Tantric (Sanskrit): literally meaning "of the thread" or "weave," it is an ancient esoteric tradition or philosophy of India that emphasizes employing personal experiences of the body and mind in ordinary household life toward the aim of self-realization, instead of the path of the renunciate who gives up his or her family, job, possession, and pleasures in search of the ultimate truth.

Transcendental meditation: a form of mantra or sound meditation developed by Maharshi Mahesh Yogi

Ujjayi (Sanskrit): translated as "victorious" breathing, this is a technique of breathing where the resistance of the air passage is increased by constricted the glottis, a part of the larynx or voice box in the throat, such that a wavelike sound is generated while breathing. Ujjayi breathing results in an energized and relaxing experience.

Upanishad (Sanskrit): elaborations and discussions of the Vedas.

Urdhva- (Sanskrit): a prefix that indicates upward.

Vairagya (Sanskrit): dispassion or detachment.

Vayu (Sanskrit): Vayu is the wind god in Indian mythology. In the context of yoga, vayus are energetic components and compartments of prana or the "life force." There are five vayus in the human body with distinct energetic qualities and locations. The practice of yoga allows one to be able to regulate the vayus through their focused awareness.

Veda (Sanskrit): derived from the root vid- which means "to know," veda literally means "knowledge" and "wisdom." However, it refers to the large body of religious texts written in Sanskrit, originating in ancient India. There are four main Vedas: Rigveda, Yajurveda, Samaveda, and Atharvaveda.

Vedanta (Sanskrit): literally translated as "the end (anta) of the Vedas," Vedanta is one of the six principle philosophies of India. Vedanta applies to the Upanishads and to the school that arose out of its discourse.

Vibhuti (Sanskrit): several meanings of vibhuti are prevalent. In the context of the yoga sutras, vibhuti means great power that is attainable through the dedicated practice of yoga.

Viniyoga (Sanskrit): term translated as "use" or "application."

Vinyasa (Sanskrit): derived from the Sanskrit term nyasa, meaning "to place," and the prefix vi, meaning "in a special way."

Vira (Sanskrit): brave.

Yama (Sanskrit): in the context of yoga, yama is the first limb of the eight-limbed path of yoga, and it refers to ethical observances for healthy living. According to the Yoga Sutras, there are five yamas: ahimsa (nonviolence), satya (truth), asteya (not stealing), brahmacharya (restraint), and aparigrapha (non-possessiveness).

Yoga (Sanskrit): literally translates as "yoke" or "bind" and is interpreted as the "union" of breath, body, and mind.

Yoga Nidra (Sanskrit): also known as yogic sleep, a practice that elicits deep relaxations while remaining alert and conscious.

Yoga Sutras (Sanskrit): an ancient text on yoga, written by Patanjali sometime between 500 BCE and 400 CE.

Yogi (Sanskrit): masculine, a practitioner of yoga.

Yogini (Sanskrit): feminine, a practitioner of yoga.

Directory of Resources

BOOKS AND ARTICLES

American Psychiatric Association. (2013). *Diagnostic and Statistical Manual of Mental Disorders* (5th ed.). Arlington, VA. https://doi.org/10.1176/appi.books.9780890425596.dsm05

Bryant, E. F. (2009). *The Yoga Sūtras of Patañjali*. New York: North Point Press.

Curtis, K. (2012). Systematic Review of Yoga for Pregnant Women: Current Status and Future Directions. *Evid Based Complement Alternat Med*. https://doi.org/10.1155/2012/715942

Cushing, R. E. (2018). Military-Tailored Yoga for Veterans with Posttraumatic Stress Disorder. *Mil Med*. 183(5–6): e223–e231.

Dass, R. (1971). *Be Here Now*. Penguin Random House.

Duan-Porter, W. (2016). Evidence Map of Yoga for Depression, Anxiety, and Posttraumatic Stress Disorder. *J Phys Act Health*. 13(3): 281–288.

Gallegos, A. M. (2017). Meditation and Yoga for Posttraumatic Stress Disorder: A Meta-Analytic Review of Randomized Controlled Trials. *Clin Psychol Rev*. 58: 115–124.

Iyengar, B. K. S. (1979). *Light on Yoga*. UK: George Allen & Unwin.

Kaivalya, A. (2010). *Myths of the Asanas*. San Rafael, CA: Mandala Publishing.

Kaminoff, L. (2007). *Yoga Anatomy*. Champaign, IL: Human Kinetics.

Lasater, J. H. (2016). *Yoga for Pregnancy, What Every Mom-to-Be Needs to Know*. Boulder, CO: Shambhala Publications.

Schiffmann, E. (1996). *Yoga: The Spirit and Practice of Moving into Stillness*. New York: Pocket Books.

Sinha, A. N. (2013). Assessment of the Effects of Pranayama/Alternate Nostril Breathing on the Parasympathetic Nervous System in Young Adults. *J Clin Diag Res*. 7(5): 821–823.

Steinberg, L. (2000). *Geeta S. Iyengar's Guide to Woman's Yoga Practice*. Vol I. Urbana, IL: Parvati Productions.

Stephens, M. (2012). *Yoga Sequencing. Designing Transformative Yoga Classes*. Berkeley, CA: North Atlantic Books.

ORGANIZATIONS

The International Association of Yoga Therapists. https://www.iayt.org
IAYT promotes yoga therapy education, training, and research, and the professional development of its members.

Iyengar Yoga National Association of the United States. https://iynaus.org
IYNAUS promotes the art, science, and philosophy of yoga according to the teachings of B.K.S. Iyengar. In addition to the national association, there are twelve independent regional Iyengar yoga associations throughout the United States.

Yoga Alliance. https://www.yogaalliance.org
Yoga Alliance® is a nonprofit that promotes and supports the integrity and diversity of the teaching of yoga through registration, setting quantitative standards, and providing scholarship programs and benefits.

WEBSITES

Core power yoga: https://www.corepoweryoga.com
In addition to providing online yoga classes and teacher training courses, this website offers a blog with information on practical topics such as poses you can do at your desk, meditation 101, self-care strategies, and even how to clean your yoga mat.

Elephant journal: https://www.elephantjournal.com
This online journal publishes on sustainable lifestyles, green living, ecofashion, and contemplative arts and offers a section of yoga with regularly updated personal stories written by yoga teachers and yoga students.

Gaiam: https://www.gaiam.com/blogs/discover

This is an online store where you can find all things yoga such as yoga apparel, props, mats, and an array of articles on how to use the props effectively and other practical tidbits.

Green yoga: https://www.facebook.com/greenyoga

This is Facebook group that offers online classes and a supportive community for yoga students and all things ecofriendly.

Martha Stewart's site with over 100 pages on yoga: https://www.marthaste wart.com/1504586/health-and-wellness

Although largely popular as a health and wellness website, the site includes over a hundred articles on yoga-related topics, including popular yoga schools and special sequences such as partner yoga workouts.

MindBodyGreen: https://www.mindbodygreen.com

Essentially a health and nutrition website, the site also provides detailed articles on yoga with emphasis on their health benefits as well as information on therapeutic yoga sequences.

Mountain soul yoga: https://mountainsoulyoga.com

A boutique yoga studio offering in-person and virtual classes in Vinyasa, Yin, and Restorative yoga, this site also offers video articles on yoga practice sequences, stress relief, and ayurvedic prescriptions that help student live in rhythm with their environment.

Yoga journal: https://www.yogajournal.com

A popular journal for all things yoga, this site offers thousands of articles on the yogic method, interviews with students and teachers, and in-depth articles on yoga philosophy and answers questions from readers.

Yogadork blog: http://yogadork.com

A blog and yoga store, this site offers articles on the latest yoga news with wit and wisdom.

Yogapedia: https://www.yogapedia.com

A comprehensive yoga encyclopedia with illustrations, instructions, cautions, and benefits on a range of yoga poses along with the Sanskrit names and classification of the yoga pose.

Index

Abhyasa, xxvii
ADHD (attention-deficit/
  hyperactivity disorder), 29–31
Adho Mukha Dandasana, 8
Adho Mukha Shvanasana, 8, 80
Adho Mukha Virasana, 8, 33, 108
Adrenal fatigue, 32–33
Adrenaline, 27, 32, 33, 103
Agnisar Kriya, 31
Ahimsa, xxvii, 17, 26, 54
Aims, of yoga, xxv
Alignment, 15, 16, 22, 24–25, 28, 31,
  34, 35, 50–52, 55, 56, 59, 63, 68,
  69, 73, 77, 82, 83, 84, 89, 90, 91,
  94, 95, 104, 105, 106, 107, 114
Amygdala, 36
Anusara, 18
Aparigraha, 26
Approach, 63–65
Asana, xxv, 3, 7
Ashtanga, 15
Astheya, 26
Attention, xxi, 6, 17, 23, 24, 28,
  29–32, 35, 48, 50, 55, 56, 61, 69,
72–73, 76, 79, 82–84, 98, 105,
  110, 111, 115
Aum, 7
Autonomic nervous system, 36, 58
Ayurveda, 78

Backbends, 8, 28, 34, 43, 61, 62, 70,
  80, 86, 88, 91
Baddha, 8; Baddha Konasana, 28, 33,
  35, 41, 51
Balance, 23–27; case study,
  101–103; mental, 25; physical,
  24; spiritual, 25; work-life-
  balance, 23
Bandha, 70
Bhagavad Gita, 4, 14
Bhakti, 14, 15, 17
Bhastrika, 10, 28
Blood pressure, 10, 22, 28, 32, 33,
  55, 56, 108, 111, 121, 123
Body weight, 22, 40, 44, 45,
  82, 92
Brahmacharya, 26
Breathing, 9–11, 69–71

Calm, 35–37
Cerebral cortex, 30, 36
Chakra, 6
Classes, 71–73; assists, 81–84;
    clothes, 77–78; frequency, 75–77;
    obstacles, 93–94
Classification, 13–18
Clinical trials, 18
Cognition, 31–32
Concentration, 4, 9, 27, 30, 31, 38
Consciousness, 6, 9, 19, 99, 100
Cortisol, 30, 32, 33, 113
Cramps, 22, 75, 106, 108, 113

Dangers, xxvi
Definition, yoga, 3–4
Dehydration, 50, 53
Depression, 19, 23, 26, 29, 32, 33,
    37, 41, 56, 57, 80, 81, 103, 108,
    113
Desikachar, T. K. V., 12, 18
Diabetes, xvii, 19, 42, 109, 111
*Diagnostic and Statistical Manual of
    Mental Disorders*, 114
Diaphragm, 70
Diet, 53–54, 78–79; Ayurvedic diet,
    54
Digestion, 22, 27, 36, 53, 98, 108
Dizziness, 50–51
Dopamine, 29
Drishti, 24; Bhrumadhye, 24;
    Hastagrai, 24; Nabi chakra, 24;
    Nasagrai, 24; Padayoragrai, 25;
    Parsva, 24; Urdhva, 25

Eating, 22, 45, 51, 53–54, 75, 79;
    satiety, 22, 29; yogic diet, 54
Ego, 14
Electroencephalography, 33
Equipment, 89; types of, 90–91

Faith, 4
Fascia, 23, 31, 40, 92
Fears of starting yoga, 93

fight-or-flight response, 26, 32, 53, 119
Flexibility, 41–42, 62–63, 91–92
Forward bends, 28, 31, 34, 35, 43, 51,
    57, 63
Functional magnetic resonance
    imaging studies (fMRI), 36

GABA, 36, 37
Guru, 72; guru-shishya parampara, 72

Hamstrings, 60–62
Hatha yoga, 13
Heart rate, 17, 22, 38, 56, 103, 115,
    121, 123
Hertz, 30
Hot yoga, 51, 68
Hypertension, 19, 28, 37, 103, 109

Injury, 41–43, 52–62; avoiding during
    yoga, xxvii
Insomnia, 27
Intensity, xxv
Intercostal muscles, 10, 119
Inversions, 54–56; arm balance,
    43, 80; forearm balance, 55,
    82, 97; headstand, 81, 82, 89;
    shoulderstand, 28, 32, 52, 100,
    103; Viparita Karani, 28, 33, 35,
    54, 55
Ishvara Pranidhana, 121
Isometric, 19, 61, 97
Iyengar, B.K.S., 12, 15, 25, 42, 67, 68,
    69, 74

Jivamukti, 17
Joints, 49–50
Jois, Pattabhi K., 12, 15, 16, 69

Kapalabhati, 9
Katha Upanishad, 4
Knee, 85, 86, 96, 103
Krishnamacharya, 12, 16, 70
Kumbhaka, 70, 100
Kundalini, 15

Learning, 31–32
Low density lipoprotein, 19
Lower back pain, 33–35

Maharshi Mahesh Yogi, 6, 123
Malasana, 38, 80
Manana, 5
Mantra, 30, 113
Massage, 23, 40, 62, 70
Medical studies, xi, xxi, 18–19
Meditation, 3, 5–7, 9, 13, 14, 16,
    17, 19, 24, 27, 29, 30, 31, 33, 40,
    75, 85–87, 99, 102, 103, 108, 111,
    113–114, 120, 122–123
Memory, 31–32
Menstruation, 56–58; case study,
    106–109; and endometriosis, 58
Meta-analyses, 18
Metabolism, 10, 22, 44, 53, 88
Misconceptions, xxv–xxvii
Mudra, 98–100
Muscle strength, 42–44, 52–53

Nada, 17, 121
Nadi Shodhan, 28
Namaste, 6
Niddyasana, 5
Niyama, 10

Om, xxv, 6–7, 30, 121–122
Online classes, 71, 93
Origins, 11–13
Oxygen, 30–31, 32, 51

Padmasana, 29, 84–86, 99
Pain, 47–49
Patanjali, 15, 17, 22
Pelvis, 16, 33–35, 57, 61, 70,
    86, 90
Post-traumatic stress disorder
    (PTSD), 113–114
Posture, core, 97; while sitting, 95;
    while standing, 95; while walking,
    96

Practice: beginning, 74–75; growing,
    74–75; maintaining, 74–75; place,
    88–89; sequencing, 78–81; time,
    87–88
Prana, 54, 57, 58, 78
Pranam, 6
Pranayama, 9, 85, 87, 111;
    breathing techniques, 9–10;
    Chandrabhedana, 28; Ujjayi, 9,
    28, 123
Pregnancy, 37–39; case study,
    109–112; pre-natal yoga, 18
Props, 15, 17, 33–34, 42–43, 55, 59,
    68, 75–76, 90, 92, 107, 110
Pulse rate, 22

Ramakrishna, 12
Randomized control trials, 114
Relaxation, 9, 25, 35, 38, 40,
    48, 53, 57, 59, 62, 68, 89, 113,
    119, 125
Religion, 4–6

Sacroiliac instability, 35
Sacrum, 83, 90, 95
Sanskrit, 6–9
Santosha, 26, 64, 92
Satya, 26
Saucha, 26
Scientific basis, 18–19, 21–23
Self-restraint, 26, 59
Self-study/Svadhyaya, xxv, 5, 55
Sense organs, 4; withdrawal, 25, 27
Sexual harassment, 84
Shaivism, 18
Shastra, 17
Shavasana, 25, 28, 33, 35, 40, 81, 103
Shishya, 72
Shivananda, 17, 67
Shravana, 5
Sideway stretches; Anantasana,
    35; Parshva Konasana, 8, 24,
    35, 43, 45
Sitting, 84–87

Sports, 39–41; case study, 103–106
Strength, xv, xxv, xxvi, 3, 15–17,
    19, 21, 22, 39–44, 47, 49, 51–52,
    55–60, 62–63, 69–70, 74, 82, 92,
    98, 102–111
Stress, 32–33
Supernatural, xxv, 5; vibhuti,
    xxv

Tantra, 6, 18
Tapas, 26, 92
Teacher, 73–74
Transcendental meditation, 6
Transformation, 22, 92
Trataka, 31
Trauma, case study, 112–115
Twists, xxvi, 8, 24, 25, 28, 34, 35, 40,
    41, 42, 59; Jathara parivartanasana,
    28, 35, 103

Ujjayi, 9, 28, 123
Upanishad, 4

Vairagya, xxvii
Vayu, 57
Veda, xxvii, 124
Vedanta, 17, 124
Viniyoga, 17
Vinyasa, 28, 33, 44, 59, 68
Vivekananda, xxvii, 12

Weight loss, 44–45

Yama, 15, 54, 124
Yoga: acro, 18; aerial, 17; aquatic, 17;
    chair, 18; definition, 3; hasya, 18;
    nidra, 28, 33, 102; power, 16, 28,
    33, 44, 59, 68, 73; prenatal, 18;
    restorative, 18, 28, 44, 45, 51, 68;
    Sutra, xxvii; therapy, 16–17, 32,
    60, 68, 113; Vinyasa, 15–16, 28,
    33, 44, 59, 68, 106, 124; Yin, 16,
    28, 44, 68
Yogi, 4
Yogini, 4

About the Author

Anjali A. Sarkar is a scientist, artist, writer, and yoga teacher. Trained in yoga since childhood under the guidance of her mother, classical Kathak dancer and yoga teacher Bharati Roy-Sarkar, and her uncle, yoga teacher Dayal Roy, in India, and later in Iyengar Yoga under the guidance of John Schumacher, Doerthe Braun, and other teachers at Unity Woods in Bethesda, Maryland, Anjali did her 200-hour RYT training from Skyhouse Yoga in Silver Spring, Maryland. Anjali is a biologist with a PhD in molecular biology and genetics from the University of Calcutta in Kolkata, India, and over a decade of laboratory research experience in biochemistry and neuroscience. She currently works as a scientist in neurobehavioral research, a science writer and editor, and yoga teacher.